Your Child's Voice

A Caregiver's Guide to Advocating for Kids with Special Needs, Disabilities, or Others Who May Fall through the Cracks

Cynthia Lockrey

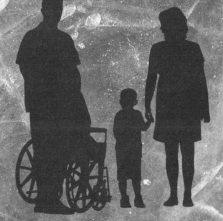

Self-Counsel Press
(a division of)

Internation

Self-Counsel Press acknowledges the financial support of the Government of Canada for our publishing activities. Canada

Printed in Canada.

First edition: 2018

Library and Archives Canada Cataloguing in Publication

Lockrey, Cynthia, author
    Your child's voice : a caregiver's guide to advocate for kids with special needs, disabilities, or others who may fall through the cracks / Cynthia Lockrey. — 1st edition.

(Healthcare series)
Issued in print and electronic formats.

ISBN 978-1-77040-304-8 (softcover).—ISBN 978-1-77040-496-0 (EPUB).— ISBN 978-1-77040-497-7 (Kindle)

    1. Parents of children with disabilities. 2. Parents of developmentally disabled children. 3. Child rearing. 4. Parent and child. I. Title. I. Series: Self-counsel healthcare series

HQ759.913.L63 2018   649'.15   C2018-903312-6
                                                    C2018-903313-4

Self-Counsel Press
(a division of)
International Self-Counsel Press Ltd.

Bellingham, WA   North Vancouver, BC
USA   Canada

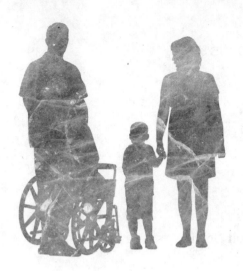

Contents

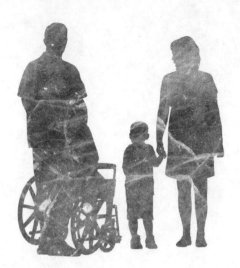

Notice to Readers

Laws are constantly changing. Every effort is made to keep this publication as current as possible. However, the author, the publisher, and the vendor of this book make no representations or warranties regarding the outcome or the use to which the information in this book is put and are not assuming any liability for any claims, losses, or damages arising out of the use of this book. The reader should not rely on the author or the publisher of this book for any professional advice. Please be sure that you have the most recent edition.

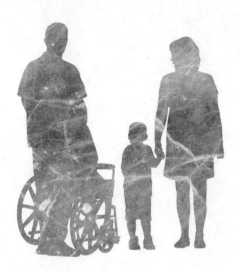

Dedication

I dedicate this book to my parents Ken and Phyllis Lockrey, who taught me the power of a parent's love and the importance of advocating for change. They have been advocating for my brother John's care for more than 40 years, long before patient advocacy was a movement. They have been honest with me about the struggles they faced at a time when parents didn't have a voice. They have also been there to listen to my frustrations about the challenges of raising a child who has medical needs. It has been a great support knowing they truly understand what my husband and I are going through.

This book is also dedicated to all the parents, caregivers, family members, medical staff, and friends who play an active role in supporting children with medical conditions. No one should undergo this journey of patient advocacy alone.

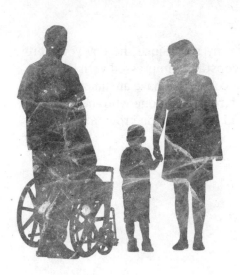

Acknowledgments

A big thank you to my husband, who is walking beside me in this life. He is an equal partner in advocating for our son, filling out applications, running to the school for meetings, and giving me his perspective on some of the roadblocks we encounter.

Thank you to my daughter for being an amazing big sister. She is a watchful eye over her brother in the playground at school, is his role model, and his best friend. She is also never shy about telling me when I need to pay more attention to her, which I sometimes need to hear.

There are so many incredible doctors, nurses, and therapists who have helped us, and continue to help us, along this journey. Dr. Renato Natale is the obstetrician who watched over me during my bumpy pregnancy, and brought my son into the world. Dr. Igor Nedic, Dr. Tom Rimmer, and Dr. Jeanne Odendall have not only kept a watchful eye over my son, but have also been a constant support for my husband and I throughout this journey.

I also want to acknowledge all the parents and caregivers I've encountered along the way. Thank you for sharing your stories, letting me cry on your shoulders, and reassuring me that I'm not alone.

Most importantly, thank you to my son. Since the day you were born you have been a fighter. I am constantly impressed with how you face adversity and how far you have come. You have an amazing sense of humor and bring a smile to the face of everyone who meets you. I am so blessed to be your mother and to watch you grow. You are definitely worth fighting for.

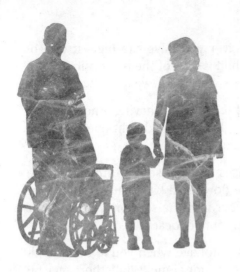

Preface

I wrote this book at the prodding of friends who have listened to my patient advocacy stories and told me they wished they had the strength to advocate for their children. Many of the people I've talked to while writing this book have said they haven't advocated in the past, as they didn't think their voice would be heard. Or, because they felt intimidated by doctors and specialists.

I realize that the term "patient advocacy" means different things to different people. It can also be overwhelming, intimidating, and a barrier unto itself. My hope in writing this book is to take some of the mystique out of patient advocacy and give caregivers some practical advice and tools so they can advocate for their children.

This isn't about becoming a champion fighter, not taking no for an answer, and becoming yet another roadblock to your child's care. Rather, it is about realizing the role you play in your child's journey and supporting him or her along the way.

Instead of being intimidated by medical staff, realize they have a role to play in caring for your child, as do you. Each person who is involved in your child's care is a member of their support team, with some members having bigger roles to play than others.

As your child's parent or caregiver you have the biggest role of them all. And advocating for your child is part of the responsibility you have in caring for your child.

As you read this book, I would recommend having a notepad beside you to scribble down your thoughts or to highlight questions you want to ask your child's medical team.

I've also included some exercises and questions throughout the book (they are also available on the download kit if you want to print copies), to help you dig a little deeper into the support you and your child will need on this journey of patient advocacy.

If there is one takeaway I want you have when you're done reading this book, it is to know that you are not alone. While there may be some lonely days in your journey, please know there are other parents and caregivers who are feeling the same emotions and have encountered similar roadblocks or challenges.

Don't be afraid to share your frustrations, fears, and successes with your friends, family, medical team, and other parents. It is through sharing our stories that we can help each other and make real change.

I wish you the best of luck in your journey of not only advocating for your child, but also raising your important human being.

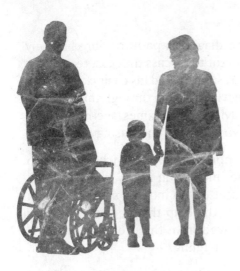

Introduction

Welcome to the club of parents and caregivers who are raising a child with medical, developmental, physical, and/or mental needs above and beyond the "norm." While the spectrum of needs from child to child is broad, and the challenges vary, what is common is the emotions and frustrations parents and caregivers face as they make this journey with their child.

The purpose of this book is to share with you some knowledge and advice from not only a parent who is making this journey, but also insights from other parents, medical providers, and educators. My hope is as you read this book, you will build the confidence to know that you can advocate for your child as well as pick up some tools to help you along the way.

My hope is also that it will open up conversations with your friends, family, and medical support team. If a certain point resonates with you, put the book down, make some notes, and take the time to talk out your thoughts with someone on your support team.

Too often we put on a brave face and don't let those around us truly know the struggles we are facing, the range of emotions we are feeling, and, most importantly, how they can help our child and us in this journey.

When we first embarked on the diagnosis path for our child, my husband and I met with our family doctor to discuss the most recent test result. The doctor put down the test results, pulled his chair closer to us, looked us in the eyes, and said, "We will love him through this." I often reflect on those simple words of advice and this message has helped me through many rough days of advocating for and raising my son.

This same doctor has also been open in telling me when I need to reach out for help. When I'm in the thick of an issue, exhausted and emotional, he will tell me not to forget to tap into my support system and not only ask for help, but accept the help that is given. It seems like simple advice when you're removed from the problem, but, it is hard advice to follow when you are struggling.

As you read through this book know that you are not alone. There are many parents and caregivers feeling the same emotions, struggling with similar challenges, and feeling they are alone in this journey. Patient advocacy is not just about fighting for your child, but also about building up and being part of a community; a collection of voices that can make a bigger change.

How big your community is and how many voices can speak together will depend on your child's diagnosis or needs, where you live, and your personal situation. Do not dwell on how loud of a voice you can make, but rather how best you can work with others to speak up and voice a concern. It is a much less isolating journey if you have people to walk beside you and support you and your child.

For some of you, this book will be the first step on this journey. Others may be further along the path in advocating for a child. What we all have in common is our love and commitment to supporting our children as we make this journey together.

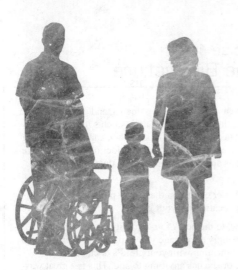

See the Big Picture: Understand Your Child's Needs

The first step in advocating for your child is to take a step back and look at the big picture. This can be a very challenging and emotional step. It is basically taking a snapshot of who your child is at this moment and summarizing what you know about his or her needs and condition. This includes listing any challenges (examples: speech delay, hearing loss, behavioral issues), summarizing any diagnosis, as well as creating an inventory of his or her treatment and medical support team (family doctor, speech therapist, occupational therapist). I have included Exercise 1 for you to work through as you read this chapter, in the book and on the download kit if you'd like to print it.

1. Start to Think about Your Child's Support Team

It is important to realize that advocating for your child is a team sport, not individual competition. As dedicated and passionate as you may be about your child, you will need a medical team supporting you in this journey. Their letters, referrals, and recommendations will be valuable resources along the way. Like every team, your child's support

Exercise 1
Looking at the Big Picture

It is very important you are clear on your child's current needs, assessments, and gaps. Too often as caregivers we feel like we are running on a treadmill of tests and assessments, focusing on going from appointment to appointment, without taking the time to step back and look at the big picture. While some children are fortunate to have a primary medical provider be the one to take the step back and look at everything, too often tests and assessments are evaluated in isolation from each other.

This exercise is designed to help you obtain better clarity on the bigger picture, which will provide the foundation for getting support and advocating for your child.

The first step is to answer the questions below, to the best of your ability. To ensure you don't leave out any important information, I'd strongly encourage you to print this exercise from the download kit, fill in your answers, and book a meeting with your child's doctor or pediatrician to review your answers and ask if he or she has anything to add. This is a great way to open a conversation about the big picture, as it relates to your child, instead of focusing on individual needs and assessments. It will also help identify if there are any gaps that need to be addressed.

For the first few questions it is important to try to remove the emotions and frustrations. While these have their place, at this stage you are looking at the facts. However, recognizing our emotions play a key role in raising children, the last questions focus on your challenges and frustrations.

What support has your child received in the past?

- Specialists

- Assessments

- Therapies

What worked?

What didn't?

What support is your child currently receiving?

- Assessments

- Therapies

Is this support sufficient for your child? What's working? What's not?

What challenges are your child currently facing?

What support do you think he or she still needs?

- Specialists

- Assessments

- Therapies

What challenges are you and/or your family as caregivers facing?

What support do you and/or does your family need?

Any emotions you want to share? Be specific on the emotion, what it is, why you are feeling it, and any recommendations to resolve this emotion (if necessary). Example: *I am feeling frustrated with delays in getting assessments. Need medical provider to follow up on where my child is on the waitlist or provide suggestions on how to advocate for improving the process.*

team is made up of a team captain (pediatrician, specialist, or family doctor), first-string support (doctors, dentist, therapists) as well as second-string support (doctors, therapists that are seen infrequently). Collectively these team members will play key roles, at different times or all together, in helping you advocate for your child.

2. Identify Your Case Manager

Once you've created this overview, ask yourself whether it is clear who the team captain or case manager is for your child. Often this is a pediatrician, but it can also be a family doctor or a specialist. It is very important one person is reviewing your child's tests, diagnoses, and updates, analyzing the information and looking at your child as a whole.

Your child's case manager is someone you can sit down with and review your observations, concerns, and needs. He or she will play a crucial role in referrals to specialists; ordering tests and assessments; overseeing prescriptions and potential interactions; as well as writing letters to get support or services for your child. While family doctors can be a good resource, too often appointments are short and related to a specific issue (ear infection, illness). Your child's case manager should be someone who offers longer appointments and reviews your child's case on a regular basis, not just when an issue arises.

When my son was a baby and toddler, our family doctor was our main contact and our visits were often done in triage mode. Although he was an incredible doctor, our appointments were spent dealing with the constant ear infections, illnesses, and individual issues (referrals for speech therapy, allergist, and the like). Since we were getting great care, and our doctor hadn't identified any concerns, we thought everything was fine. It wasn't until we moved to a new community in a different part of the country that our son was referred to a pediatrician with the intention of looking at his hearing loss and speech delay. In our initial meeting, our pediatrician, who has since become our son's case manager, took a holistic look at our son and began ordering a number of assessments, as she had a fresh approach and wasn't bogged down in triage mode.

Over the course of our first year with this pediatrician, our son had a long list of assessments, tests, and treatments. All of these results and reports were shared with our pediatrician as well as our family doctor. This process allowed our pediatrician to have a better understanding of the broader challenges facing our son, and find some connections. Every three months we met to review the findings and discuss the next steps. While it was a long process with as many as nine specialists and frequent tests, the end result was a clearer understanding of our son's challenges, and ways to get support for him, as well as defined next steps.

Our pediatrician is the one person besides us who knows the big picture and serves as a resource for our son's other doctors. She continues to play a key role on our medical support team. She is someone who is on our side and we often count on her to support us when we need to advocate for our son.

As with all relationships in life, it is important your case manager is someone you connect with and trust. If you don't have mutual respect and trust, your child won't get the support needed. While this relationship will take time to build, you also need to listen to your gut instinct if you feel friction. Any friction between the caregivers and case manager will only create another barrier in helping your child.

A case manager is the most important person on your child's medical team. This is the person you will lean on the most, likely shed a few tears with, and to whom you will express your frustrations and share your successes. He or she will have a comprehensive understanding of your child, and will be privy to much personal information. For these reasons, it is crucial your case manager sees you and your child as people and individuals versus just patients and is willing to stand beside you and advocate for your child when needed — every time — without question. See Exercise 2 (also available on the download kit).

A Pediatrician's Perspective
Dr. Dominique Eustace
Mother of three school-aged children

My vision is to have medical providers come up with responsible options and offer them to the family. The family can then direct which treatment option or intervention they want to tackle first and share how their family or community can implement them. For this to happen, the family needs to be honest with me throughout the process on any barriers or challenges on their end.

Questions to Ask Your Case Manager

Your case manager will play a key role in your journey with your child. For this reason, you need to make sure you have a mutually respectful relationship and determine who is best suited to fill the role of your child's case manager. Is it a pediatrician, family doctor, nurse practitioner, psychologist, or another specialist? There are many options available.

It is important you have a discussion with the person you've identified as your child's case manager to ensure he or she is prepared to take on this role. Don't assume because your child has a pediatrician that this person sees himself or herself in the role of your child's case manager. In some cases, he or she may assume your child's family doctor is the case manager. This assumption could result in no one assuming this role.

If one medical professional doesn't work, don't give up until you find someone who understands your child and his or her needs.

Here are some discussion points and questions to ask a potential case manager.

We are looking for someone to take on the role of case manager for our child. This means one medical professional who will review all of his or her tests and assessments, not just the ones you request, but also requests from other physicians and therapists involved in our child's care. We are hoping you, as our child's case manager, will be the person to take the step back, look at the big picture and help identify any gaps or concerns. We are also asking that you provide the continuity of care, reviewing any reports or assessments, and helping us advocate for our child, when needed.

- What do you see your role being in supporting my child?
- Do you feel comfortable or agree to be our child's case manager?
- What does that role look like for you?
- How long will our appointments be with you?
- How often will we meet with you?
- Can we call you if we have questions outside of regular appointments?
- Do you have privileges and/or work shifts in the local hospital?
- If our child is admitted to hospital, will you be treating our child or will it be another pediatrician on call?
- If you won't be treating our child in hospital, will you still be monitoring his or her case? Can we call you if we have questions or need support when in hospital?
- Do you want to be included on all test results ordered by other doctors?
- How often will you review our child's file with regard to any new results or reports?
- How will you interact with other members of our child's medical team, including family doctor, dentist, specialists, and therapists?
- What role do you see yourself playing in our child's development and support requirements?
- What role do you see me/us as caregivers playing?
- Are there rules we need to follow (this can include having tests done in certain timeframes, ensuring the case manager is included on all test results)?
- What role do you see yourself playing in advocating for our child?
- Can we call on you to write letters, attend meetings, or to follow up on referrals?
- If so, how much time do you need to prepare these items?
- If we run into challenges along the way, how will you support our child and us as caregivers?
- What are the limitations of your involvement?

Doctor's Job

The role of a doctor is to provide medical leadership for the family. The parent is the child and family expert who knows the family's resources and limitations.

Communication to the rest of the medical team needs to come from the medical lead. This person is often the pediatrician or family doctor. While some parents may want to take on this role, it's better if they allow their doctor to do this.

Sadly there are times when no one is taking lead and the family needs to step up. When this happens, it is important as a parent that you push back and be clear on the role the team leader is to play.

If there is friction or differences of opinion between the parent and doctor, it is worth having an honest discussion with your child's doctor to explain your differences and see if you can resolve them. If this can't be done, ask if he or she can recommend another doctor who is a better fit. You should be able to say "Look, I don't feel comfortable with what you've said. I'm worried about my child and I need you to help me understand why are you doing this."

It is important doctors have honest conversations about the treatment. If you switch to longer feeds, your child might vomit less but then you might have fewer hours free off the feeding pump. This change might not make the child or family days easier even if it makes the symptoms better. Doctors need to give families the option of doing less such that they can enjoy their child and family.

Parent's Role

The role of the parent is to be the expert on his or her child — how the disease, disability, or diagnosis uniquely affects the child. This includes being aware of how the child's symptoms might look, which can be different from the textbook definition. The parent also needs to be the expert on how the disease or diagnosis impacts the entire family.

An example is if you have a child who doesn't do well with morning appointments, it is important you make sure your medical provider understands the challenge associated with early appointments instead of taking the time given and not getting to the appointment.

While part of a parent's role is to be in tune with his or her child — knowing when something is off — the parent still needs to let the medical team make the diagnosis and propose treatment options. I have seen parents come in, say their child's color was off, and state, "I think it's a urinary tract infection and he needs septra." Although the parents' diagnosis may ultimately be correct, it is still important to allow the doctor to take a full history and assess clinically to ensure no other issue is impacting the child.

There is another risk if families assume the role of the medical expert. The families that are documenting the seizures, medication doses and time, may be so burdened with tasks or so focused on disease management that they miss normal family time. They note the number of seizures not the number of smiles.

Community Resources

As a pediatrician who has moved from a large urban center with a children's hospital to a rural community, I see the disparity in resources for children. The further a patient lives from a large urban center, the fewer the resources available. This is especially true for children with chronic disease.

This can be a delicate conversation to have with a family. The family must fully understand the choices available to them and implications associated with their decision.

The medical team should ensure informed consent. The medical team shouldn't assume what is best for the family. The parent should be aware of all the options, especially when there is the potential that access to these resources could make a difference in the child's life. Depending on the child's needs, keeping the child in a smaller community could place a higher care burden on the family, as there are fewer funded supports available. Inversely, moving to a community with more resources can mean greater financial burden and social isolation for some families.

Final Thoughts

Parents or families are key to delivering effective pediatric medicine. Parents need to be the voice for their child. Parents should not be afraid to speak out for what works best for their child. It is also okay for parents to ask and ensure their child's doctors are talking to each other. Finally, if you find resources that help your child, don't be afraid to share this information with your family doctor and/or pediatrician.

3. Establish Your Medical Team

Now that you've established your case manager and developed a relationship, it's time to build the rest of your team. These people will play an important role in helping advocate for your child. If you're further along in your journey and have a well-established medical team, great. However, if you're still working through your child's diagnosis, have moved to a new community, or are struggling through the process, it is important you are clear on what individuals make up your child's medical support team and the role each of them will play. Who are the lead players? These could be key specialists or therapists. Now who are the supporting players? Be as clear as you can on each individual involved in your child's case, the role they will each play and how they can provide support if issues arise.

Too often when roadblocks or challenges arise, parents and caregivers get frustrated, curse the system, and throw up their hands in frustration. By taking the time to determine who is on your medical team and the role each member will play, you'll realize the depth of people you can call on when needed. I would recommend going through this process when things are calm, so you can take a detailed inventory versus reacting in an emotionally charged situation. This will ensure you don't overlook key supporters, and that you follow up on the opportunity to discuss ways your child's medical team can support your child before an issue rears its head.

As mentioned with your case manager, when inventorying this group, be clear on whom you have developed personal relationships with, where you have mutual respect and trust, and who has the best understanding of your child and his or her needs. These are the individuals you'll want to lean on first, as they will know you are taking an active role in advocating for your child, not just complaining.

It may seem odd or uncomfortable to see your case manager as a person versus medical provider, but personal relationships will allow for frank discussions when facing roadblocks. You need to break down some of the patient/doctor walls, so doctors can truly understand your family as a whole and its associated needs and struggles.

See Exercise 3 (also available on the download kit).

4. Potential Tests

As you work with your team to understand your child's needs and get or manage a diagnosis, there are no shortage of tests and assessments that may be conducted. This is not meant to be a comprehensive list, but rather some of the more common tests for you to discuss with your medical team:

- Hearing test
- Speech assessment
- Occupational therapy assessment
- Physical therapy assessment
- Blood tests: celiac markers, iron levels, vitamin deficiency, thyroid, complete blood count
- Urine or stool test
- Autism spectrum disorder
- Developmental assessment
- MRI, CAT scan, and/or ultrasound
- Antinuclear antibody test (ANA) to detect autoimmune diseases
- X-rays

As a parent who has watched a child go through many of these tests and assessments, know that while this can often be a long, exhausting, and somewhat frustrating journey, it is an important part of getting an accurate diagnosis for your child. Don't give up but rather work with your child's team and know you are helping your child. Yes, you may be tired of driving from appointment to appointment, but each test and assessment plays an important role in helping your case manager see the big picture. When it comes to advocating for your child, you will need to rely on these tests and assessments to help state your child's case for needing support. You will look back and be grateful for the amount of analysis that went into your child's diagnosis and/or treatment plan.

Once your child has received a diagnosis, I encourage you to move on to Chapter 2.

Exercise 3
Setting up Your Medical Team

When setting up your child's medical support team, it helps to take a page from organized sports and fill in the positions below accordingly.

Team captain (case manager)

This is the main person overseeing your child's case.

First-string support

This can include your family doctor, specialists who play an active role in your child's case, and key individuals providing treatment (speech therapist, dentist, physical therapist). These are the people who know your child as a person versus a name on a file, and sees them on a regular basis.

Second-string support

Included in this list are supporting specialists you see infrequently (neurologist; ear, nose, and throat specialist), and individuals who provide assessments not treatment (occupational therapist, behavioral therapist). Your child may not have regular interactions with these individuals but they hold a piece of the puzzle.

Potential team members

Pediatrician

Family doctor

Nurse practitioner

Dentist

Ear, nose, and throat specialist (ENT)

Neurologist

Allergist

Urologist

Gastroenterologist

Internist

Physiologist

Psychologist

Psychiatrist

Speech language pathologist

Occupational therapist

Physical therapist

Behavioral therapist

Mental health counselor

Other: _____

Other:_____

Dr. Joey Dahlstrom
Mother of three school-aged children

Understanding Roles

The role of the parent is to link your child's health professionals. Unfortunately, there is no communication between the medical community and dentists unless the parent links them. Typically, once linked, the dentist will get copied on the specialists' reports written for the family doctor. Depending on your child's needs, this could be important in his or her overall care.

If this linkage isn't made, there is no communication between practioners, dentists may not understand the full scope of the child's condition and may not treat appropriately or ill-prepare the family for the child's future dental needs.

The parent also has a four-step role to play in his or her child's care:

1. Prevention: Assisting with tooth brushing with fluoridated toothpaste and flossing, providing a low sugar diet, and taking your child for regular checkups.

2. Seeking appropriate practitioner care early and planning for future dental needs. Whether orthodontics or restoring missing teeth, this requires financial planning.

3. Avoiding projection of your own dental anxiety onto your child as this serves to only heighten your child's anxiety.

4. Communicating with all practioners involved in your child's care about dental concerns and asking for inter-communication from dentist to medical practitioners and vice versa.

The role of the dentist is to first take care of any immediate dental concerns: dental decay, oral pathology, and dental abscesses. Next, would be the discussion of what the future holds: return of pathology, missing teeth and outcomes, or orthodontia needs. At this point the dentist may refer to an oral medicine specialist, pediatric dentist, and/or orthodontist depending on the child's needs.

Advice for Parents

Prevention is paramount. Treating dental decay in a special needs child is challenging for all involved and may require a general anesthetic with possible removal of baby teeth. Once baby teeth are lost, the space is no longer held for the following adult teeth and they may not erupt properly. Without proper positioning, the ability to maintain the adult teeth in the years following becomes more challenging and some of those adult teeth may be lost.

It is important to have the discussion on what the future holds as early as possible with the dentist. There are certain X-rays that can be taken if the child can stand still to know what teeth are present below the baby teeth and which are missing. With that knowledge, the family and dentist can best decide the timing of treatment for orthodontic intervention, cyst removal, and other interventions as necessary.

The recommended first dental visit is at one year of age or six months after the first tooth eruption, whichever comes first. This provides the opportunity for the dentist to meet the child and vice versa but also serves as the beginning of desensitizing the dental visit.

The challenge with a special needs child can be that he or she has had many medical interventions and can often be very fearful of anyone in an office setting. Typically, if no immediate problems are detected at that first visit, the child is seen every six months.

If the child is deemed high risk for developing tooth decay, a topical fluoride can be painted on the child's teeth at each visit. Fluoridated toothpaste should be used at every tooth brushing, twice a day. Fluoride is our best defense against tooth decay. NO bottle should be given prior to bed without brushing afterwards. Breastfeeding should also be followed by brushing with a fluoridated toothpaste.

Currently, all dentists trained in Canada learn to see patients at that first year or six months after the first tooth. However, not all dentists are comfortable seeing young children and particularly those with special needs. If that is the case with the parent's own dentist, I would recommend the child seeing a pediatric dentist. Parents can self-refer to the pediatric dentist, so no referral from a general dentist is required.

Cost can be a significant factor. In some communities, medical costs are covered for low-income families. It's important you research any support available in your state or province.

Pitfalls to Avoid

The main pitfall to avoid is Dr. Google. This may serve to only increase the parent's anxiety about the child's condition and often provides erroneous information and treatment recommendations. It may also tick off your child's medical team if you are basing decisions for treatment on anecdotal information versus evidence-based treatment.

Limitations in Advocating

The limitations with advocacy could be geographical — not everyone has access to specialists that typically reside in major cities. In certain communities some dentists may not be receptive to patients' needs or desires to recommend care from a specialist. Another limitation could be financial — dentistry is often privately funded — only a small percentage of people qualify for government funding, where available, which is typically based on family income, not severity of need.

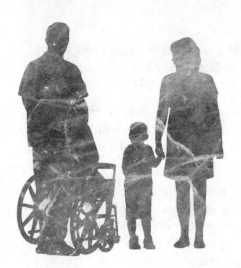

2
The Diagnosis

Some of you reading this book may already have a clear diagnosis or diagnoses for your child and have picked up this book to help you understand and improve your role as your child's advocate, while others are still working your way through this process. Regardless of where you are in the journey, realize that tests, diagnosis, and treatment can be a recurring loop. As children develop, new issues may arise and previous challenges may no longer be as relevant. It is often left to the caregiver to be on top of his or her child's progress, track changes, and advocate for new or repeat testing as the child develops.

That being said, once you have your child's diagnosis (and in many cases multiple diagnoses) it's important you clearly understand what this means for your child as there is no one-size-fits-all diagnosis. You need clarity on whether or not there is a main diagnosis (such as genetic deletion or micro deletion) and secondary diagnosis (low muscle tone, speech delay, seizure disorder), which relate to the main diagnosis. Sound confusing? It can be. That is the reason why you need to work closely with your child's case manager to be clear on the various diagnoses; to minimize confusion and help to understand how the diagnoses relate to each other.

While we as parents and caregivers often cringe at hearing labels, since we don't want our children to be seen as labels, it is important we are clear on the terminology, and what it means for your child specifically. Clarification helps us begin to understand and see the big picture, and use the labels to get the support our child needs.

Without the labels, roadblocks are harder to remove and you are often left feeling isolated and alone. Labels can come with a community of support, and give a name to a situation you've been struggling to understand.

For example, for years, autism was a little understood disorder. Children did not receive the treatment and support needed. These children were often seen as difficult, slow, or mentally challenged. Children now labeled with autism, receive more specialized care and treatment, and caregivers become part of a community of support.

For those of you who have children without the now common labels of autism or attention deficit hyperactivity disorder (ADHD), to name a few, it is equally important to have a diagnosis for your child, whatever that diagnosis might be.

When my son was first diagnosed with low muscle tone, it was a term I had never heard. However, when I began doing research, the puzzle pieces fell into place. I finally had a diagnosis and description of challenges he was encountering. The diagnosis and associated label enabled me to have informed conversations with his medical team and advocate for the specific support he needed. On this journey I learned swimming and therapeutic horse riding were key therapies to help build his core strength. The label helped me find programs and have discussions with his instructors about his specific needs. This was incredibly rewarding as I finally felt I was playing an active role in helping my son, now that I knew how to explain things. Labels can play a crucial role when advocating for specific support for our children.

At the same time, labels can be overwhelming and confusing to understand. Two children sharing the same label can be on completely different ends of the spectrum. This is why trying to understand a label through Google searches is a dangerous exercise. It is human nature to focus on the worst-case scenario. It can be hard to take your eyes away from the doom and gloom to really understand a label in relation to your child. Labels also need to be understood in reference to your child's bigger picture. Is low muscle tone or speech delay the main label/diagnosis or a secondary label related to the main diagnosis? Where is the priority in therapy and support? Can therapies be integrated to address various labels?

When my son was a toddler, he took speech therapy in a swimming pool. While it may seem odd, the swimming kept his muscles occupied, making it easier for him to focus on the speech therapy, since he finds it challenging to sit in a chair for long periods of time.

In this scenario, the pool-based therapy was at the recommendation of the speech therapist. But sometimes it falls upon the caregiver to get creative and work with the support team to find ways to integrate therapy that not only helps your child but also will be something he or she will enjoy.

1. Getting Organized

Once you have your child's diagnosis, reports, and assessments, it's important you get everything in writing. While it is standard practice for your case manager to have copies of his or her files and other specialists' in your child's file, you should ask for copies for your own files.

Keeping an organized record of results at home will come in handy. Trust me. Remember, you aren't analyzing these reports, but rather keeping a copy for your records after you have discussed the results with your case manager. It is also good to have a copy of reports in case you want to refer to or share them with any potential new team members. These reports are often beneficial for schools to review in either developing an independent education plan and/or understanding behavioral issues.

Through my advocacy journey for my son, my binder filled with reports has been my secret weapon. I have the reports organized based on the doctor or therapist. When we were strongly advocating for an educational assistant at school (more about this in Chapter 3) my husband and I relied heavily on this binder. I became very familiar with the contents of each report, photocopying reports which best backed up our case for why our son needed an educational assistant, and using the labels as a means towards getting the support we knew was necessary for his success.

Without written reports, we would have been left trying to summarize his needs and attempting to paraphrase assessments, which would have been viewed as our opinion versus the observations and conclusions of unbiased professionals. The reports added much needed validity to our observations as parents.

In a system where funding for support is limited, it often falls upon parents and caregivers to clearly identify the need for support by putting together a tight package of reports, letters, and assessment that cannot be disputed. Sadly, the children who don't have this package often are left receiving little or no support, despite their needs.

I have also learned the value of sharing reports with other key members of my son's medical team (first-stringers). When we go for tests or assessments, I make sure not only the doctor ordering the test, but also the relevant team members, get a copy of the results as it could be weeks or months before I see the doctor who ordered the test. In our case, since I see our son's pediatrician and family doctor on a regular basis, I'm often able to review reports with them, getting their thoughts and insights. It also helps these individuals see the big picture versus just their piece of the puzzle. This is beneficial when you are asking them to advocate for your child. If they are only aware of their piece, they won't be able to see how their piece relates to the big picture.

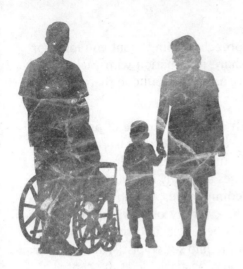

3
Get Support

Armed with your child's diagnosis, now comes what is often the most complex and challenging step: getting support. This is the step where your advocacy skills will be honed and tested, often repeatedly. This is also where the legwork discussed in previous chapters will be invaluable. Before you can advocate for support for your child, you must clearly understand your child's diagnosis and needs so you can identify the gaps. The relationships you have developed with your child's medical team will also be called upon throughout the process of getting support.

The support your child requires will be based on his or her specific needs, which can be related to any diagnoses and conditions. The support needed can include physiotherapy, occupational therapy, speech therapy, educational assistant, mental health counseling — the list goes on.

For some caregivers, their child's case manager will have some clear recommendations on therapy and support as it relates to the main diagnosis and primary needs. Others will be left trying to piece together the puzzle on their own, or through discussions with a number of members of their child's medical team, each looking at their own specific pieces of the puzzle. This approach, an often frustrating experience, can result in therapy done in isolation versus taking a holistic approach in addressing the collective needs of the child. If you find your child caught up in this approach, it's important you look for ways for the various therapists to share information with each other. This could include you photocopying a report from one therapist and sharing it with other team members.

Accessing these therapies, which can be a mixture of private and publicly funded, depending on where you live, will also depend on your child's age and condition(s). In many areas, children not yet in school have access to different therapies and early intervention services than school-aged children. In some communities, therapy is offered at shared resource centers that provide a variety of services for young children under one roof. This system is beneficial to caregivers, as it allows you to have a discussion with your child's therapist(s) about other services your child could access that may be available at the center.

Before my son entered school, he was receiving speech therapy at a shared resource center. His case manager then referred him for occupational and physical therapy assessments, also at this center. This was extremely helpful as we were able to share results with each of his therapists, which then resulted in the therapies they provided being modified to meet needs identified by other therapists. The therapists also discussed his case with each other, as well as the best ways to engage him in therapy. They quickly learned he saw their games as a way of getting him to do the therapy. They modified their collective approach so my son was able to select what he wanted to do each session, making him feel that he was in control versus being told what to do by the therapist. At the end of the day he still received therapy, but on his terms. This approach was shared with new therapists to ease the transition of working with my son.

Through discussions with his speech therapist, we were also made aware of other services our son could access, including what I call a "fly on the wall" visit to his daycare. This visit involved a woman from the center spending a few hours over three days quietly observing our son at daycare. He wasn't aware she was there watching him and recording his interactions. To our son, she was just another adult in his classroom. I shared her observations with many members of his support team, with each finding the information important insight into how my son behaves in a comfortable environment, versus the often sterile and clinical settings of doctor appointments or assessments. This was helpful, as my son had learned that staying quiet and not participating in tests and appointments was how he could have power in situations he didn't want to be in. Not ideal when he was having a developmental assessment.

This observer's report was particularly beneficial for his autism assessment. At this appointment he put his non-cooperation superpower to the test, responding to as few questions as possible. Once again, not ideal. However, the assessor had previously read the observer's report, which summarized a number of interactions he had throughout the day with his classmates at daycare. It was this report, combined with his positive body language toward his dad, which led to the conclusion he did not fit on the autism spectrum.

We would never have been aware of this "fly on the wall" assessment opportunity if it hadn't been for conversations with his speech therapist. We had talked to her about how we were trying to determine what support our son would need when he started school. Therapists are often tuned into the bigger system, and by sharing your concerns or frustrations; they can help offer solutions or connect you to other resources that may be available.

1. In-School Support

Once children enter school, they may be eligible to receive therapy by therapists paid for by the school or school board. The challenge here is these therapists often have heavy caseloads, and therapy is either limited to a few minutes a week or left to the classroom teacher to implement. This is only if you or your child's support team has advocated for him or her to receive the necessary therapy and it is available in your school district.

If your child has received therapy prior to entering school, it is important you work with these therapists to advocate for your child to continue to get support in school. In many communities, therapists know each other, and it isn't difficult for them to send an email or pick up the phone to talk to another therapist about your child's case. That is, if you ask. This isn't something they will naturally do, as they are busy managing their own workloads. For this reason, it is important you ask for their help in providing an overview of your child's needs and advocating on his or her behalf for in-school support. Your child's therapists will also be able to share reports, work plans, and other information that will make the transition to school-based therapy and entry into the classroom an easier one.

To be clear, in-school therapy support is not the same as getting an educational assistant (EA), teaching assistant (TA), or teacher's aide (TA) for your child. The term for this in-school support with special needs varies between countries. However, what is common is getting support is its own battle, one about which its fighters can tell you war stories, and show you battle scars.

When we were preparing for our son to enter kindergarten, we had the option of two public schools: one French immersion (which is publicly funded in Canada) and the other our local public catchment school. We ended up selecting the French immersion school, despite our concerns about the extra layer of learning, because of the responsiveness and support offered by the administrative staff. Even with the clear understanding by the principal and resource teacher that our son would benefit from an educational assistant (or teaching assistant), it was an uphill battle to build a case for a child who did not have the labels commonly associated with the allocation of additional classroom support.

Our son was sent for an autism assessment, as an autism diagnosis would be a good label for getting him this support. When the assessment came back that he was not on the autism spectrum, we were back to the drawing board (although happy to have one less label to add to his file), as this diagnosis would have secured an educational assistant (EA). In trying to argue the case for my son to have an EA, my husband and my parent advocacy skills were tested to the limit.

The initial intake meeting to register our son at the school and discuss his specific needs (with the goal of stating a case for him needing an EA), involved a room full of people, including the principal, vice-principal, resource teacher, kindergarten teacher, speech therapist, special needs intake advisor, my husband, son, and me. We had 30 minutes to provide an overview of our son, his needs, and state our case for his needing additional support in the classroom. All this while our son was pretty much ignored and left to play with toys in the corner of the room (even though we had been told it was essential he attend this initial meeting).

We had been given only a few days notice to prepare, not enough time to include his case manager or members of his medical team in this meeting (which is something I'd highly recommend). At the 30-minute mark the next parent and child were waiting at the door, so our meeting abruptly ended.

To say this was a frustrating experience is an understatement. While everyone involved was kind and supportive I was left feeling it was up to me to compile the information to support his case for an EA.

The resource teacher also told us that the end result would likely be that he would not receive support due to the limited funds available for EA support in elementary schools.

In discussions with my son's case manager, as well as his therapists, I knew early intervention and support was crucial to his transition and success at school. Despite our binder full of reports (which I had shared with his school), it was still left to me to establish a bulletproof case that the school could present to the school board to support the funding request. I was left having to create this case while trying to raise two young children and work a full-time job.

Being Type A personalities, and determined to get our son the support we knew he needed, my husband and I accepted the challenge and began working as a team. My husband called our son's therapists to get copies of missing reports (we hadn't started the binder at the beginning of our journey). I met with his case manager (pediatrician) and was clear on what I needed documented in a letter from her to the school board, asking her to include as many labels as possible. We also called each of his specialists, getting them to supply letters outlining the importance of early intervention and list labels related to their piece of our son's puzzle. Many of these phone calls involved lengthy discussions about how best to relate his needs in the letter to meet the requirements of getting an EA.

All of this was being done against a very tight timeline put on us by the school. We had about two weeks to compile the relevant reports and letters before the school board met to review EA funding and staffing allocations for the following school year. Talk about pressure. After many in-person meetings, phone calls, and emails, we had developed a thorough package outlining our son's diagnosis and associated needs. A month later the principal called us to let us know our parent advocacy paid off — our son had qualified for an EA for September. Phew. When I asked how he qualified for full-time support, when we had been told to expect minimal support, the principal said it was due to the bulletproof case we had created. The various letters and reports from a variety of doctors and therapists had made it impossible for the school board to turn down our request for an EA, as numerous professionals had clearly stated the need for support.

As I celebrated our success, I began thinking about what happens to the children whose parents are not able to or don't understand how to advocate on their child's behalf. How many years and frustrating experiences at school does it take for these children to get the support they need to be successful or enjoy the school environment?

In talking to teachers, I've learned that more often than not children enter school with needs that are obvious to the teacher, but either the parents are unaware of these needs or the child has not yet received the testing and diagnosis required to support an EA. In these situations, it can take many months, even years, for the school to work with the caregivers and medical support team to get the testing and diagnosis the child so badly needs. As some of the tests involved have long wait lists, the child is left struggling in the classroom, often becoming frustrated, disengaged, or deemed a problem child, all because he or she does not have the necessary support to help him or her succeed.

So why does this happen? In some cases a child that seems rambunctious as a preschooler is now a disruptive student in the classroom. An experienced teacher may recognize the child as having ADHD or another condition that impedes his or her learning, and the lengthy process of getting testing and diagnosed begins. Other times the parent has sensed his or her child has challenges, but doctors have dismissed his or her concerns. It isn't until the child enters the classroom and is compared to other children the same age, that the parent has access to the resources and support available through the school to begin advocating for the necessary testing.

Sadly, in other situations the child is labeled as difficult or challenging and shuffled through the school system grade after grade, never getting diagnosed and provided with the support that would help him or her be successful. This child often becomes disengaged with school, acts up in the classroom, and leaves high school as early as possible. Unfortunately, in some cases the support a child receives depends on the school he or she is in, the experience and personality of the classroom teacher and how strongly his or her caregiver advocates on his/ her behalf. In countries without a publicly funded medical system, the financial ability of caregivers to pay for their child to visit doctors and have tests and assessments done can be a limiting factor in the child's diagnosis and subsequent documentation needed for the child to qualify for in-school support.

While it may seem unfair that the squeaky wheel gets the support, and children who don't have people advocating on their behalf are left struggling, unfortunately in an overtaxed educational system, this is often the case. This is why it's so important for caregivers to have a clear understanding of their child's needs and work with their medical team to advocate alongside them not only in the early years but also throughout their school days to ensure the medical team continues to review the child's needs and associated support available.

The more information you can have in writing the better. Schools love written reports, letters, and test results. Teachers and principals want what's best for each individual student, as well as the classroom as a whole. However, they must also work within their budget. Educational assistants or teaching assistants are hard to come by due to the extra costs. Because of this, the school and caregivers must create the bulletproof case requesting support that I mentioned earlier.

This is also the time to call on every member of your medical team to be in your corner and lend his or her voice of support. They each hold a piece of the puzzle and now's the time for them to put their piece on the table, helping the school see the bigger picture of your child's needs. If possible, have them attend a meeting at the school with you or call the principal to explain your child's case. At a minimum have them write a letter with their specific recommendations, with the case manager providing a letter outlining the bigger picture, bringing all of these individual recommendations together. Having a conversation with each team member ahead of them writing their letter will help ensure the individual letters all meet the specific needs of your child.

See Exercise 4 (also available on the download kit).

An Educator's Perspective
Dwayne Wessel
Teacher, consultant, university instructor in the
Masters of Education program
Father of two high-school-aged children

The Parent's Role

Parental involvement is the key to a student's success. Parents need to know their input and advocacy in their child's education drives the team toward effective outcomes. I remember sitting in an independent education plan (IEP) meeting and a parent telling the team, "I know that I might not be popular at the end of this meeting but I did not come here to be popular. My job is to advocate for my child and make sure that my family's needs are understood. The decisions we make will affect my child long after they leave your school setting. I would like to get along with all of you by the end of this meeting but that is not my mission today." That statement stood with us throughout the meeting and has stuck with me throughout my career.

One piece of advice I have for parents is to take videos of your child as he or she develops and to capture his or her progress. This way you will be able to look back and see how far the child has come, which will help you with perspective during the difficult times. Your child's progress will spike and sometimes plateau but it will never stop. I remember a mentor telling me, "never move a mountain at a time, sometimes you move it a pebble at a time."

The Teacher's Role

Effective teachers have the ability to check their attitudes at the door. Education degrees are not something to hide behind during a disagreement with a parent. Degrees provide information to share with parents, not to shut the parent down. The teacher should see himself or herself as someone who implements the team's decisions rather than someone who overrides or trumps the input of others. A teacher cannot be right alone. Accepting input and seeking guidance from parents is not a sign of weakness; it is an indication of professionalism.

Advice for Parents

Know that you are not alone. Each journey is unique but there are consistent paths. Other parents and staff have gone through the process before and can provide guidance. I have met parents who make it their job to make sure that other parents will not face the same struggles as they have. When you are starting out, seek those parents for support and advice. As you gain more experience, become one of those parents for people who are starting their journey.

Some points to remember:

- Do not spend a lot of time apologizing for your child's actions.

- Do not go into meetings alone.

- Have grownup chairs at meetings. Don't allow meetings to be set up like the last supper with the administration on one side and the parents sitting alone on the other side.

- Do not forget to send your child's team a card during the holidays to say thank you.

Pitfalls to Avoid

Do not think that your role as an advocate and/or parent is a popularity contest. You will get into disagreements with staff and that is sometimes a part of the process. Avoid becoming so upset that you come across as unstable. In the past, I have had to consult for parents who were no longer allowed on school property.

If you'd like to discuss your child's progress, ask the teacher when he or she is available to talk instead of trying to talk to him or her during instructional time. Use phrases like, "I am concerned that this did not get done," rather than, "why didn't you do this?"

Some common ways parents tick off teachers is by only pointing out the negative things that have happened; accusing others of not doing their job; being inconsistent; agreeing to implement strategies but not following through; and constantly going over the teacher's head to administrators.

The Risk of Not Advocating

In the past, I have seen parents who have not advocated for their child. Often, but not always, as a result, the child's goals become less of a priority, his or her behavior plans are less likely to be followed, and his or her performance tends to stagnate. Teachers are humans with busy workloads and without regular meetings, updates, and support it sometimes becomes difficult for many of them to keep on top of an independent education plan [IEP]. This is why it is important to check in regularly with your child's teacher, to ensure the plan is being followed and issues addressed. Keeping the two-way flow of communication open between the teacher and the parents will benefit everyone involved.

Active versus Passive Involvement

An active role to me is a parent who is there in the good and the bad, someone who can hear bad news without pointing fingers, and who emails often to celebrate his or her child's success. A passive role is someone who does not speak during meetings, reply to emails, or ask for updates.

I do not judge parents for being in either of these roles. I know that some parents are overwhelmed; some have more time than others, while other parents need support to feel empowered as well as know they are a welcome and essential part of the team. To help support the whole student, a teacher needs to be there for the whole family, through the good and the bad.

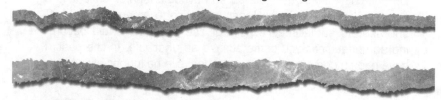

A Mother's Perspective
Tammy Isaachsen
Mother of two school-aged children

The Early Years

For the first couple of years after my son was born, my focus was on advocating for his medical needs. A lot of my time was spent educating medical professionals in our small town about his condition: achondroplasia. Although this is the most common type of dwarfism, it is quite rare (1 in 25,000–40,000 births). I had to become an expert on his condition, and worked with medical professionals on helping them understand the importance of my son being referred to specialists who had experience treating other children with his condition.

If you're not in a large city with a children's hospital and you have a child with a rare condition, you will also need to become the expert on your child's condition so you can advocate on his or her behalf and ensure he or she gets the medical care that is necessary.

I was lucky to find a local pediatrician who was willing to learn alongside us. Even though she'd never had a patient with achondroplasia, from day one she said let's figure this out together. In connecting with other parents, I know this can be the most challenging part, finding a doctor willing to take on that role and truly understand the unique needs of children with rare conditions.

School Years

As my son ages, the challenge I now face is transitioning from being his voice to encouraging and helping him become a voice for himself. Adding to this challenge is my son's quiet and reserved personality.

I'm trying to be his microphone; giving him the opportunity to speak up for himself when he needs something at school and repeating it back in a louder voice if needed.

Since my son doesn't have behavior or learning challenges, which are generally the more typical special needs in schools, it has been difficult educating teachers and administrators on his unique needs. Due to his short stature, he has a number of physical limitations and can easily be overwhelmed and nervous in a busy schoolyard. It has become a balancing act between me advocating on his behalf to get the support he needs at school and helping him find his voice as well as gaining the confidence to speak up while he's at school.

I've spent a lot of time at the school advocating for his needs. And I believe he wouldn't have received an educational assistant (EA) if I hadn't strongly advocated for support. I know without his EA and my ongoing advocacy, he would struggle with more accessibility challenges. I'm in the school visually seeing issues and speaking to staff to accommodate his needs.

If a parent isn't actively involved, the child will fall through the cracks. Our schools are so full and busy, and your child isn't the only child who has needs. Sadly, if I wasn't the squeaky wheel, the coat hook wouldn't have been lowered to his level or the soap placed in the bathroom where he could reach. These are issues that are not on the radar of teachers. If you aren't speaking up for your child's needs, he or she will go to the bottom of the list.

As a caregiver you need to recognize there is a strain on resources and the school is busy constantly putting out fires. If you aren't at the school either voicing your concerns or helping your child speak up, your child may be lost. It's important to take the time to visit the school, talk to the classroom teacher and administration, as well as have an active role in supporting your child and identifying issues.

Community Connections

As a parent, what I've found most beneficial is connecting online to different groups within the dwarfism community. Through the connections I've been able to learn more about the challenges facing these individuals, everything from the baby years to school age challenges and into adulthood. I've also learned about the assumptions that are often made regarding abilities based on the physical appearance of individuals with achondroplasia. Many of these assumptions are not accurate.

The connections I've made have been vital in learning more about my son's condition and being able to talk to people who have been there and done that. I definitely wouldn't be where I am now on this journey without these connections.

Our family endeavors to regularly attend meetings and social events, and sometimes larger conferences that bring together individuals and families with dwarfism. Although it can be expensive and challenging juggling family life, it has been a huge benefit to my son. It's incredible watching my son's spirit rise as he walks into a hotel full of people who have the same condition instead of being the minority in a school with 450 children.

By making these connections he's able to see he is part of a bigger community. The friendships he makes will continue to help and support him as he grows.

My son has a condition I don't have. I recognize he's part of a whole other culture and world. He's walking and living an experience much different than mine. Taking the time to attend these events is a huge step in helping him feel included versus excluded.

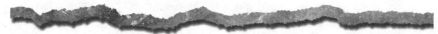

2. Ongoing Communications

There is so much effort that goes in to getting an educational assistant or teaching assistant, that too often when caregivers have succeeded in securing this support they think all is well and take a step back. While receiving in-school support of any kind is a big relief, it is just the first step in establishing ongoing two-way communications with the school.

Exercise 4
Developing the Case for an Educational Assistant/Teaching Assistant or Additional Support

As mentioned earlier, it is important you ask for a meeting with your school prior to your child entering kindergarten (in the early spring prior to your child starting school). If your child is already in school and encountering challenges, you can ask for this meeting at any time during the school year, but recognize that funding allocations might only be made once a year.

What is important is you come as prepared as possible to meetings and have the ammunition needed to back your case for asking for additional support for your child. Be clear on the support you feel your child needs. Is it an educational assistant/teaching assistant, speech therapy, personal education plan, other specialized support, or a combination? While this meeting won't resolve the issue, it will be the first step in an often lengthy process.

Here are some items to bring to the initial meeting:

- Copies of all assessment and reports (speech, physical and/or occupational therapy, autism assessment, hearing tests). You may need to ask your child's therapists for a report specifically related to identifying needs and recommendations for the classroom environment.
- Test results: Any results that could impact your child at school.
- Diagnosis: If your child has multiple diagnoses, your case manager will need to write a letter summarizing the main diagnosis and related secondary diagnoses. In some cases this will involve a request for support from a variety of professionals, not just the classroom teacher. You'll also need letters from each specialist involved with your child. The more letters you have, the stronger the case you will create for support for your child.
- Report cards: Any issues identified by previous or current classroom teacher, relating these issues to findings from assessments, testing, or diagnosis. You want to clearly make the connections between known challenges, reasons for these challenges, and the case for providing additional support to help overcome or minimize these challenges.
- List of medications: Any medicine that needs to be administered at school either on a regular basis or in the event of an emergency.
- Summary of your child's needs: As the caregiver, what do you see as his or her main needs? What support do you feel your child requires? Are there times in the day when more support is needed (e.g., recess, lunch, gym class)? Is he or she better in the morning? Afternoon? Does the child have difficulties transitioning between activities? What upsets him or her? What helps to calm him or her down?

Questions to ask during your school meeting:

- How many students will be/are in the classroom?
- How many of these students have identified needs?
- How many students in this classroom receive additional support? (Note that in some school boards/districts there is a limit to the amount of children with additional needs per classroom. This is why it's important to know how many children in the classroom have identified needs and/or are receiving support.)
- What resources are currently available at the school? (Resource teacher, quiet space, speech therapist, modified gym classes, etc.)

- How can my child access those resources? What information do you need from me to help him/her access those resources?

- Can I have a meeting with the appropriate individuals who provide these resources?

- How many educational assistants/teaching assistants are allocated to the school? How many children do they support?

- When is funding allocated for educational assistants/teaching assistants? Can additional support be provided mid school year?

- What additional information do you need from me?

- Would a meeting or phone call with my child's case manager be helpful?

- Are there any additional assessments you would recommend for my child?

Following this meeting, here are some possible next steps for caregivers:

- Supply missing copies of relevant reports, diagnoses, or assessments.

- Follow up with an email to the principal after the meeting summarizing what was discussed, reports/letters provided, and agreed-on next steps (it is important to have an electronic record of conversations).

- Call the principal or appropriate staff member, one to two weeks after the meeting, to see if he or she needs any additional information from you. Ask about the status of any requests for more information made at the meeting.

- If your child does not receive the support requested, meet with the principal to determine why not, and explore opportunities to appeal this decision. Then follow up with your case manager to identify next steps (if appropriate).

- If your child does receive support, meet with the principal to establish regular meetings with the individuals supporting your child to get progress reports and identify any challenges. Don't wait for a problem to happen. Be proactive and continue to have a presence in the school. How often you attend meetings will depend on your child and his or her specific needs.

It is important to be seen as a resource and member of your child's team versus an obstacle. How you interact with the school in the early stages will set the tone for interactions throughout your child's school years. Try to be positive and professional, but also clear on the support your child requires with well-documented needs. Although it can be challenging, try to limit your emotions and focus on the facts. It is the facts that will get your child support, not yelling, crying, or getting upset. Although it can feel good at the time, getting upset can result in the school seeing you as a problem parent, and negatively impact future interactions.

Notes:

I learned this lesson the hard way. As mentioned earlier, my husband and I threw ourselves completely into the task of creating a case for our son to receive an educational assistant. When he started kindergarten, we had the initial meeting with the school administrators and various resource support providers to develop his individualized education plan (IEP). A month after this plan was developed, I was called back to the school for a meeting to review the plan and his progress to date.

I was completely underprepared for this meeting. I had gone alone, as my husband was home with the kids (the meeting was held after school dismissal). I wasn't prepared for the amount of people who would be in this meeting, including the principal, resource teacher, school board resource supervisor, speech language pathologist, my son's educational assistant, the kindergarten teacher, and a couple of other administrators who were involved in his case. As they went through his IEP, they would stop and ask me my thoughts on various aspects of the plan. We had 30 minutes to go through this plan, for me to provide on-the-spot input and have any modifications made.

If this wasn't stressful enough, throughout the meeting, the various individuals around the table who worked directly with my son provided their observations of his first month at school. Some of these observations were very difficult for a mother to hear. Yes, I knew my son had some challenges (hence his need for in-school support) but in the back of my head I'd always hoped I was overreacting. To hear educational professionals say things like "severe delay," "socialization issues," or "difficult to understand" made me want to curl up in a ball and cry my eyes out.

This is the difficult part I want to share with you if you've never been through one of these meetings. If you have, you know my pain. Somehow, you will need to find a way to deal with all the emotions coming at you while still being able to process factual information about your child. This is why I'd highly recommend you never attend these meetings alone. It is important you bring your spouse, a relative, or a friend with you. This way as you are hearing information that brings you to tears, your support person can answer the questions and continue on with the meeting.

For me, I spent part of the IEP meeting in a daze. I remember actually thinking "it's okay, you can sit and cry about this later. But for now, answer their questions." Somehow I managed to get through the meeting, yet I know I likely missed part of the discussion and didn't answer all of their questions.

My second piece of advice about ongoing communications is don't assume the IEP is being followed to the letter. The classroom is a busy place with a number of teachers and support resources involved in your child's education. As such, your child's IEP may not always be followed as written.

A few months after the IEP meeting I just mentioned, we received a phone call from our son's teacher very upset about his behavior. She told my husband he had been acting out in class, not listening, and not respecting his educational assistant. After my husband hung up the phone, he thought about what he had heard, with some of the concerns being uncharacteristic for our son.

Before we spoke to our son, my husband and I discussed the phone call and tried to figure out what was causing this behavior. Was our son getting enough sleep? Was he not feeling well? Then we began wondering if he was being given the opportunity to eat throughout the day versus at set snack times (as per his IEP).

I emailed the resource teacher and his classroom teacher with questions aimed at further understanding the root of their concerns. Many of these questions were basically asking if identified areas in his IEP were being followed. Turns out they were not. The resource teacher (who oversees his IEP) had not been informed of the classroom teacher's concerns, his educational assistant did not know our son needed regular snack breaks (as he had joined the team mid-year), and other items of the IEP were not being followed. This resulted in a second IEP meeting, with the same team as before and his new educational assistant, to review his progress and remind everyone of the items contained in the IEP. In setting up the meeting I made sure it was held during school hours so both my husband and I could attend. No more attending meetings by myself, trying to hold it all together.

I also learned I needed to have more of a presence at the school. Even though my son normally takes the bus, at least twice a month my husband or I will drive him to school or pick him up so we have a chance to chat with his educational assistant and/or teacher in person. We've also bought a notebook we keep in our son's backpack, to communicate with the school instead of writing notes in his lunch that may or may not get read (depending if they get lost in his backpack).

You too will learn lessons along the way and find solutions that work for you to keep the lines of communications open with the school. But when challenges arise, it's important to not take it personally or get upset. Remember your child is one of many children who are demanding attention or have special needs. It is understandable that errors may be made, that's why it's so important to keep the lines of communications open and have a physical presence in the school so you can have conversations before there is a problem.

3. Navigating Waiting Lists

In many communities, the amount of children needing support greatly outweighs the number of trained professionals and support providers available. Waiting lists can be long, which is especially challenging where early intervention is key.

Depending on the size of your community, your financial situation, and amount of insurance coverage, private therapy is an option you may want to explore. While private speech and occupational therapy can be expensive, it can also help a child get much needed support while he or she waits weeks or months for publicly funded therapy, if it's available. Your family doctor, pediatrician, or school can provide you with a list of private therapists in your community.

If your child needs physical therapy, ask what his or her therapy requirements are, and about alternatives to traditional physical therapy. For my son, the timing of his publicly funded physical therapy session conflicted with his speech therapy, with no alternate time slot available. So, I had to weigh which was more important. Deciding that speech therapy was the bigger priority, I arranged a phone call with the physical therapist to discuss other options available. She recommended swimming and therapeutic horse riding as the best activities for his low muscle tone. She also advised me that we needed to make these activities fun for our son, rather than have him see them as therapy. She explained that if he enjoyed these activities, he would more likely continue them for life. If at any point he wanted a break, we needed to respect his wishes, as he would be more likely to return after his time away versus being forced to continue in therapy he wasn't enjoying.

Our physical therapist also provided specific recommendations for his swimming and riding instructors. This ensured he truly received the program that was best suited to his needs and his condition. While there were costs to both programs, the local pool and horse barn also offered subsidies to low-income families.

Don't be discouraged from looking for private therapy based on your family income, as there may be financial support available. If you have a YMCA in your community, it offers affordable membership options, which can be adjusted based on your family income.

A Speech Language Pathologist's Perspective
Lisa Dymond
Runs a private practice and provides in-school support

When I'm working with a new child, it is important to know right at the beginning the role the parents or caregivers is willing to play in their child's speech therapy. Are they willing to spend 10–15 minutes a day working on speech at home or do they want to limit their involvement to taking the child to weekly speech therapy sessions?

Where the rubber meets the road in terms of a child's progress is how involved the parents are in their child's therapy outside of the weekly sessions.

When I'm preparing a treatment plan for a child, by having a clear understanding of the role the parents will play, I can prepare a program that will support the child as well as meet the family's needs. This helps provide role clarity for everyone and avoid frustrations.

I see speech therapy as a team approach, and we are all in it together. It is important caregivers have a conversation with their child's speech therapist about their intentions, time commitments, and level of involvement in their child's therapy throughout the treatment plan. As personal situations change, the therapist needs to be aware of any changes in home support so the child's plan can be adjusted accordingly.

Funding Paperwork

When parents are seeking private services, and they have funding through a third party, such as the Autism Funding Unit or the At Home Program, it is important for parents to be on top of the paperwork for their child. This means having a conversation with the speech pathologist about the required details before therapy can be initiated.

Typically, an authorization number is assigned that is specific to the child and the speech and language pathologist. Only then can services begin. Third parties will not pay for backdated appointments so the paperwork must be initiated, promptly. Furthermore, third parties will not pay for appointments that are missed without adequate cancellation notice.

Families need to check with their speech pathologist about the cancellation policy and be sure to cancel any appointments within that time frame, and agree to billing for missed appointments. The speech pathologist has reserved the time slot for your child, and this time needs to be respected.

Recognizing Time Commitments

One of the common challenges I encounter is a parent not considering or appreciating the time allocated for his or her child's treatment. If a child has a 60-minute session, the parent needs to decide how he or she wants this time to be spent. Does the parent wants the child to receive a full 60 minutes of therapy? If so, this means there is no time left at the end of the session for the parent to ask questions or discuss his or her child's progress. If the parent would like time set aside to talk with the therapist, he or she needs to include this time within the child's 60-minute time slot.

When parents recognize that appointments are set for a specific time, it helps the speech pathologist in sticking with his or her schedule. That means if parents show up late for the appointment, the clock doesn't start when they arrive. Rather, the therapy will be limited to the time remaining in their scheduled timeslot.

As a professional with a heavy caseload, I have a set amount of time for each child and often have back-to-back appointments. Containing sessions within the scheduled timeframe means the family who comes next will also receive the full amount of time scheduled for them. This is especially important when services are delivered in the home and I need to travel between houses.

I would strongly recommend at the first appointment parents have a discussion with their child's therapist about role clarity, time allocation, payment requirements, missed appointment policy as well as service delivery so everyone is on the same page and to keep communications clear and successful.

In-School Therapy

I've found communications with parents of children who take private speech therapy is usually good as the parent often brings the child to the appointment. Where I see more challenges is communicating with parents who have children receiving in-school support.

Since speech pathologists are traditionally not included in parent-teacher interviews, there are more barriers to communicating with parents and less opportunities to discuss a child's progress.

Many schools will allow parents to sit in on the occasional speech therapy session. Unfortunately very few parents take advantage of this opportunity. I recommend that parents try to observe a session early in the school year and again at the end of the school year, to understand progress and how to best incorporate therapy strategies at home.

If work or other demands don't allow an in-school visit, parents can also call the school and leave a message for the speech pathologist requesting a time to discuss the child's program. When parents call they need to recognize their call may not be returned immediately, as most therapists travel between schools. Rather, when leaving a message, parents should be clear they are calling to request a phone appointment to discuss their child's progress and review how they can support the child at home. This helps the therapists prepare for the phone call.

Taking the time to either attend a session or speak to the therapist would make a big difference in the child's progress, as it would ensure the parents are clear on how they can support their child and help further his or her speech development.

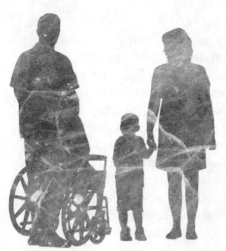

4
Identify Your Family's Needs

As caregivers we spend so much time focusing on our children's needs, that we often overlook our personal needs or our family's collective needs. If you are going to advocate for your child, it is important you take stock of the broader needs of your family as a whole as well as those of the individual members within your family, not just the one child.

1. Time with Each Individual

In my journey with my son, I have found that I can be spending a period of time so focused on his needs and advocating on a specific issue, that I forget to take my head out of the weeds and look at those around me.

During one of these times, my daughter and I were walking back from a neighbor's house. She asked me a question, and with my brain running a mile a minute, I didn't hear her so I didn't respond. That was the tipping point for her. She had a complete meltdown, screaming that I only cared about her brother and never spent time with her. She said I didn't even know she was alive and ran away crying. I stopped dead in my tracks, consumed by mom guilt. Had I been focusing too much on her brother? Even though I felt I was giving her attention, had my attention been too one-sided?

I gave her some space to cry and be upset, and then went to her room to have a quiet conversation with her. Instead of justifying that I love her and I spend time with her (which was my first instinct) I forced myself to sit quietly and asked her to explain to me what was bothering her. I encouraged her to talk about her feelings and what specifically she wanted and needed from me. I was impressed with how much she understood about her brother's needs (which we had been trying to keep from her). After a few tears and a bit more screaming, it all came down to the fact she wanted one-on-one time with her mom. She didn't want to share time with her brother, but wanted her mother's undivided attention. This is something she saw her brother getting from me but was something she thought she wasn't receiving.

After a lengthy talk, our solution was establishing mother-daughter dates. On these dates we carve out time for each other, to do something out of the house, while my husband and son have guy time. This way both kids feel like they have one-on-one time with the parent they spend less time with (or they perceive they spend less time with). My daughter and I will go for a sushi lunch, hang out at the beach, or go for a walk in the forest. It doesn't have to be a big trip or cost any money. Your children just want to spend quality time with you.

We plan these outings in advance so they become a priority, are put on the calendar, and actually happen instead of becoming something I keep promising but never deliver.

I have also found the best way to support my daughter is to ensure she has an activity that is her special time. She is a horse-crazy girl, so her joy revolves around being at a horse barn. Although riding lessons can be expensive, we've been able to find a barn that allows her to be involved in all aspects of the horses, not just riding. She goes early to her lessons to feed the horses and help with chores. This allows her to spend more time at the barn on lesson days.

She also spends half a day once a week mucking out the stalls, feeding and watering the horses, and grooming some of her favorite horses. In return for her hard work, she earns an extra riding lesson from her trainer. It's a win-win situation as she is fully immersed in the horse world and comes home happy and tired.

By allowing her to have her own special activity she knows we are supporting her in her passion. While we sometimes bring her brother with us to the barn, I also try to make sure that at least twice a month I take her to the barn on my own. I stay and watch her lesson, hang out while she feeds the horses, and take the long way on the drive home so we can have some extra time together to chat about her lesson. Being at the barn without her brother also gives me a chance to talk with the barn owners and be a part of this world that means so much to my daughter.

2. Date Nights

The other area that tends to get overlooked when you're busy caring for kids is time with your partner. This is an area my husband and I are continuously working on, as it becomes a lower priority with all the other items we are juggling in a week. As many of you will know, the challenge is finding the time and energy to go out with your partner on a date, especially if you have young children, and hiring a babysitter adds an additional cost and obstacle.

Whenever I talk to friends about some of the challenges we are going through, the usual advice they give me is to make sure my husband and I don't forget to have our date nights. Then they proceed to tell me about how they have weekly date nights with their partner. While I know they are trying to be helpful, their children are often older and have fewer needs. Or they have grandparents living locally who are actively involved in childcare, including having the grandkids over for sleepovers. Sadly, this is not a option for those of us raising children away from family support, which adds another barrier to spending time alone with our partner.

One particularly helpful conversation involved a woman telling me how important it was I get a nanny so I wouldn't be stretched so thin. When I explained my children are both in school, she said even better, the nanny can do house cleaning and meal preparation for me. When I thanked her for the advice and mentioned the financial cost of a nanny wasn't in our budget, it was obvious this reality wasn't something she could comprehend.

The point of my little rant is that while there may be challenges finding time with your partner, it is important you find your own ways to stay connected so your relationship remains strong. As you know, you need to draw upon this relationship many times during your times of advocacy and throughout your journey of raising children.

If you are a single parent, it's even more important you get some much needed "you" time. This could involve finding a friend or neighbor to walk with, enlisting the help of grandparents (if you're fortunate enough to have them living nearby), or joining a club (dragon boating, book club). You need time to focus on activities you enjoy, so you can recharge your batteries for the never ending job of parenting.

My husband and I try to go for lunch once a month on a weekday, as this doesn't involve babysitters and upsetting bedtime routines (which becomes its own barrier to getting out of the house). We spend this time talking about work, sharing schedules, talking about future projects and yes, inevitability talking about our children. The "no child talk on dates" rule becomes more of a stress than a reality. After all, they are a major element and focus of our lives.

When you have a child with special needs, there are often items related to his or her care or treatment you don't want to or should not discuss in front of your children. I learned this the hard way when we were considering adding a dog to the family. I had read about the therapeutic value of dogs and how they can help with speech delay (as kids naturally carry on conversations with dogs in a way they may not with people). One day while talking to my kids about what kind of dog we should get, my son said, "Will it help make me better?" My heart sank. What had I been saying to my husband about dogs and their therapeutic value? I wasn't aware of how much of the conversation my son had heard or understood as he was still in preschool. After that gut wrenching moment, I learned it was more respectful to have conversations about my son and his challenges with my husband on our lunch dates, away from the home. Or at least wait until both kids were in bed sleeping.

When we lived close to family, we were able to enlist their help on babysitting. Now we take advantage of their cross-country trips to see us to pop out for a quick walk or quiet supper. However, in both circumstances these were short outings as my parents are elderly and aren't able to keep up with two young kids for too long. Whatever your situation, you need to find what works for you and your family, but make sure spending time alone with your partner is a priority that doesn't get pushed to the back burner. You will need to have a strong partnership so you can support each other during the tough times.

A Father's Perspective
Kyle Yakimovitch
Father of two school-aged children

When I look back at life as a father before my child was diagnosed, there was an intuitive feeling that my child had some challenges and needed help. This was a scary time, as I didn't know where to go or what to do. It took some courage to share my concerns with my wife, as voicing them out loud made them all the more real. However, when we did finally talk, I was somewhat relieved that my wife shared my concerns.

This honest conversation started us on a journey that is ongoing. I'm glad we both recognized our initial intuition and made the decision to work together to pursue various ways of having our child assessed, diagnosed and getting the support needed. While this was a scary time, at no point did I ever feel it was insurmountable. I knew we would have to dedicate a lot of time and energy supporting our child on this journey, but as a family, we would do our best to help.

As we've gone along this road with our child there have been a number of fears my wife and I have had to deal with along the way. For me, one way I've dealt with my personal fears is to become educated on our child's challenges, diagnosis, and therapies. To me it's been important to have a good understanding of the diagnosis so I can ask the right questions or push for the appropriate resources. Having open conversations with my wife has also been a huge support.

Talking about your emotions can be a challenge for men. In those times when we are struggling with a difficult situation, I have found my strength being in focusing on the facts. It doesn't mean I'm not emotionally connected, but rather I'm the parent taking a step back and trying to look at the issues or challenges rationally.

In our times of advocacy, I've been able to lay out the facts for everyone involved. It's been a beneficial process as it's allowed my wife and I to play an active role in helping guide and steer the ship to the most efficient results. Or, at the very least, take us down the roads we needed to go without being clouded or muddied with the bombardment of information coming our way.

This has allowed us to create priority lists instead of trying to deal with all of the information collectively. By approaching challenges from a factual perspective, it's also allowed me to gain acceptance of the situation. And this is a tough hurdle to jump over as a parent.

While I've always felt we can help our child get past the obstacles, there's a part of me that wants to deny my child has a problem. When you're cuddling, playing, or spending one-on-one time with your child, you can't accept there's anything wrong with your child, as he or she is such a key part of your family. Your child is a part of you, part of your being and it's painful to digest and acknowledge that your child has challenges.

But once I accepted this fact, it allowed me to move forward and educate myself. By doing that it helped me deal with my fear, pain, and guilt and get past it. It also allowed my wife and I to connect, acknowledging we were in this together. It wasn't until the point where we both accepted our child had needs, determined what they were and the direction we needed to head that we were able to connect as a unit, which was more efficient and less emotionally draining than going it alone. There's a need to connect as parents, but for that to happen there needs to be a real focus on and agreement of what the path ahead looks like and the roles you each will play. This doesn't mean you will always agree, but what's important is you continue to work as a team while sorting through any differences.

Support

To truly work as a team, support needs to be on both sides: me supporting my wife and my wife supporting me. A big lesson along this journey has been really listening to my wife when she offers her intuition, which is a big part of the equation in supporting our child. Mothers truly have a special connection with their children, and are able to sense when they are ill or struggling. I have learned for myself this mother's intuition should be respected, not ignored.

There have been times when the journey of advocating as well as raising our child has been overwhelming for my wife. As strong and stoic as she is, I can always tell when she is struggling and having a painful time. During those moments all I can do is hold her hand, sit down, listen, and offer any support I can.

When I am overwhelmed, I listen to my wife as she shares with me the efforts she is making to advocate for our child. This offers some relief, as I know she is actively engaged to get our child the support needed. It also gives me permission to take the time I need to regroup.

Time Together

When you are raising a child with special needs, everything is so busy and there's so much time, effort, and resources put into your child and children that there is little time left for us as a couple. While it's all well and good to schedule and book dates or lunches, it's an ongoing struggle to find time to connect. Some weeks we only have minutes alone together without kids, and that's often when we are zoning out watching Netflix.

Since we have moved to the other side of the country without any family nearby, we've had to cultivate new friendships. This has been done through finding likeminded individuals with a similar family situation or at least compassionate about our struggles and understanding our needs.

I give huge kudos to my wife for her ability to create new relationships. While I lack the icebreaking capacity, her ability to make strong connections is something I really value in her. Once those friendships have been made, I truly enjoy them.

My wife has a knack for being open and honest about our situation and making meaningful versus superficial connections. She is able to read people and quickly determine who is sincere and authentic.

When my wife and I do find 15 minutes to have a quick chat or an hour for a lunch date, these are truly invaluable times. While we still talk about our kids, it's also a time where we truly listen to each other and find out what the other person needs. These are touch points of appreciating what's happening, what we need from each other, even if it's a break from the whirlwind of activity and appointments for our child.

These conversations can also be as simple as discussing what food prep needs to be done for dinner, time scheduling, finding out the biggest work pressures each of us is facing, and looking for ways we can move forward together as a team.

The time alone can also offer space to be creative as the stress of supporting our child isn't there. By taking the time to get away for lunch, we can sit back and see the bigger picture, and determine if as parents we need to change direction, continue course, or relook at things entirely with a new philosophy or new information based on the latest doctor's report. This is a difficult thing to do when you're at home with little ears listening to your conversations.

Finally, I have found a positive attitude to be the one thing that gets me through the tough days. With this positive attitude I have found each day I get stronger, even with setbacks, which can be disappointing and otherwise cause a defeatist outlook. Instead, I recognize and appreciate all the experience I have behind me and recognize the importance of continuing to march forward. For me it's about always putting one foot in front of the other as you get through the challenges, enjoy the successes, and continue to advocate for your child.

3. Create a Support System

All families need a support system, but it is especially important when your family includes a child with additional needs. Your support system will evolve as your family situation and your child's needs change. For some, your support system will be family members who live nearby. For others living away from family it can include neighbors, friends, or even coworkers. And for others it will be a combination of all three. What's important is you have a support system that is available for emotional support and can also be called upon at a moment's notice in times of crisis.

When we lived near our family, we still relied heavily on our neighbors to look after our daughter during emergencies. They were able to quickly run over and sit with her while we rushed to the emergency department. For longer term support, my parents were able to take our daughter while we spent time with our son in the hospital. We also relied on other parents to take our daughter to dance classes, pick her up after school, or have her over to their house for a play date while we focused on our son and giving him the care and attention he needed. We didn't want our daughter's childhood to be filled with memories of doctors' appointments or hospital visits. We used our support system to keep her busy and provide her with fun outings, away from the hospital.

When we moved across the country, away from family and established friendships, we had to start from scratch and develop a new support system. Thankfully this evolved naturally through relationships we formed with neighbors, coworkers, other parents, and new friends we met along the way.

The first time we had to rely on this support system was when our son had a seizure. To shield our daughter from seeing her brother in distress we sent our daughter to our neighbor's house while we anxiously waited for the ambulance to arrive. While I jumped in the back of the ambulance with my son, my husband went next door and checked on our daughter, who had willingly run to the neighbor, also not wanting to see her brother having a seizure. By the time my husband arrived, our neighbor, a grandmother and kind soul, had already immersed our daughter in a competitive game of cards, in front of a plate of treats that she was happily munching away on, having put the trauma at home out of her mind. Our neighbor greeted my husband with a warm smile and a hug, told him to leave our daughter with her and to go focus on our son. She even popped up to the hospital a few hours later to bring us something to eat and get an update on our son's condition without our daughter present.

Over the next few days, our neighbor's house became our daughter's second home and safe haven. Knowing our daughter was safe and being cared for was a huge relief as it allowed us to follow her instructions and focus on being with our son. Once his condition stabilized, our daughter was able to come for hospital visits and see that her brother and I were OK. The nurses were kind enough to include ice cream treats on these visits, so there was a positive memory associated with visiting the hospital.

Although this situation described above was spontaneous and we had to trust that our neighbor would help us during our crisis, we had never had a conversation with her about our needs and her willingness or ability to support us. Thankfully she is a straight shooter. Once the dust was settled and our son was out of hospital, she sat us down with a glass of wine and talked to us about how she could help support us. While we are often hesitant in sharing our son's struggles, she was now involved through her actions on that day and we needed her help. My husband and I filled her in on our son's medical history, what we had gone through, what we were going through, and what was yet to come. Needless to say there were a few tears involved as she was the first person in our new community to whom we had opened up and shared our story.

After getting a hug and another glass of wine, she explained exactly how she could help and what her limitations were in terms of her own commitments. She has since become a huge support for our family. She often picks up our daughter from the bus stop when we're out of town for appointments with our son or stuck in traffic. Since she's a positive, energetic person, our daughter loves spending time with her, and is often disappointed when we come to get her, telling us that we are home too soon, begging us to let her stay longer.

The abrupt and unexpected situation of our son's seizure and hospitalization also opened the door to conversations with new friends and coworkers. Once again I had been limiting how much I had been sharing with others as we had only been living in the community for a few months. I was amazed at how many people reached out to help our family. One coworker brought a much needed coffee and muffin to the hospital the morning after we were admitted, and came over with a huge pot of homemade chicken noodle soup when we were discharged. Another friend dropped off a latte and scone for me on her way to work. All without being asked.

In letting down my guard, friends and coworkers also shared stories of challenges they went through with their own children, some whom were now grown and others who are still young. One woman who shared her challenges with me has become one of my closest friends and a huge part of my support system as her son had similar struggles when he was a child. She is the person who encouraged me to write this book, as she said she never knew how to or even that she could advocate for her child when she faced roadblocks with his care and treatment. Looking back on her journey, she wishes she had the strength and knowledge to advocate for her son so she would have felt she had some control in often out of control situations. Through letting down my guard and sharing my experiences, I was able to make a connection with a mom who is there to support me during good times and rough patches.

A Mother's Perspective
Mary Dougherty
Mother of two young children

Keeping Notes

When my daughter was a few months old, I began noticing she was missing some developmental milestones and was struggling with basic tasks. I started writing down my thoughts, my observations, putting a date next to each note. As we worked through her diagnosis, these notes became invaluable as they provided a record that I could review with her doctors.

Often doctors will say, when did you first notice this or that thing happen? As a parent, memory fades, so having notes to refer to and review will help you and your child's medical team to see the bigger picture. These notes will also help your child with being diagnosed and getting treatment sooner.

A Different Motherhood

Before my daughter was diagnosed, someone said to me, "It's her journey, not yours." On one side this advice was good to hear as it reminded me she was on her own path when it came to learning to walk, talk, and reach other milestones. But on the other side, this person didn't recognize that raising my daughter is my journey, too.

This is what motherhood looks like to me; helping my daughter along her journey as she faces obstacles and deals with struggles. There is a bit of mourning that comes with my version of motherhood. I don't think I will ever get over that.

Everyone wants to have the perfect child and give them the best childhood. While my daughter is perfect in her own way I'm always waiting for the other shoe to drop. To find out what else is wrong.

It's not that my husband and I were less happy when she finally walked or used words. It's just that these moments have been bittersweet due to the struggles it took to get there. We can never fully appreciate the moment, as it didn't happen at the time it should have. And then, for a split second we're almost normal, until once again other children jump ahead and leave her behind.

Getting Support

It is important you find that one person who believes you and truly understands the struggles you are going through as you parent a child with special needs. You need someone who will be on your side throughout the journey, as you navigate through the struggles and celebrate the small successes. Oftentimes this person won't be someone from your family or existing circle of friends. He or she may be someone you meet at a support group, a paid counselor, or another parent of a child with special needs.

It is important you connect with someone who's going to believe you when you say what's happening with your child isn't normal, and whom you can openly and honestly talk to when you're having a bad day.

When my daughter was young, before her diagnosis, all of my friends and family said she was fine when I expressed concerns about her development. They made me feel crazy for thinking there was anything different about her. That was a very hard time for me.

When she was finally diagnosed with a genetic condition and related challenges, this same group said, "Oh, now we believe you." Her diagnosis confirmed I wasn't crazy and my instincts were right, but it was difficult knowing so many people hadn't believed me when I had expressed my concerns. That's why I had worked so hard to get her tested; I wanted to know my suspicions weren't unfounded. I knew something was wrong and I badly needed to find a way to support her. Finally getting her diagnosed was also a way of making our life as a family function better so we could all get the support we needed.

When I talk to someone who understands how I feel, it's like I'm part of a club that I wish I didn't belong to. But I'm also glad to have someone to talk to who truly understands my struggles and listens without judgment. There is so much value in confiding in someone who knows you aren't crazy and appreciates that your journey as a parent is a much different one from many other parents.

It also gives you the opportunity to think out loud and talk things over with someone who isn't emotionally connected but still understands the fears and challenges. Sometimes your medical support person doesn't really get the frustrations and emotions parents face, as they are not living with a child who has needs.

My greatest advice to other parents is to find at least one person who truly understands your situation and can be there to support you. While you might be tempted to put on a brave face and make this journey alone, having an ally will make the difficult days a bit more bearable.

4. Connect with Other Parents

Thankfully, I learned early on the value of connecting with other parents going through a similar journey when I was hospitalized for two months on bed rest while I was pregnant with my son. I wrote about that too, in *Bed Rest Mom* (Self-Counsel Press, 2018). Although I had previously spent three months on bed rest while pregnant with my daughter, it was a home-based bed rest and an isolating experience. However, when I was diagnosed once again with placenta previa (placenta covering the cervix) during my pregnancy with my son, my obstetrician (OB) took no chances, and sent me to a large teaching hospital more than an hour from my home.

After a few days of sitting and crying in my room wondering how I was going to get through my six-week stay, I decided to try and connect with other women on my floor. I did this by going door to door with another mom and organizing a pizza party in the common room for the other pregnant women on our antenatal (high-risk pregnancy) unit.

This was the best thing I ever did for my mental health and personal well-being. Over the next few weeks, our group of moms spent countless hours laughing, crying, sharing stories, supporting each other during difficult times, and connecting as mothers and people. Having spent one bed rest at home alone and a second bed rest surrounded by women going through a similar experience, reminded me of the importance of not only connecting with others, but more importantly, spending time with people going through a similar journey.

None of us was your typical pregnant woman, working up to our due date, having low-risk pregnancies and deliveries or heading home hours after giving birth. Rather we were a group of women with conditions that were potentially life threatening to our babies and us. We were grateful for every additional day of pregnancy, knowing that our babies could be born at any moment. Sadly some of the babies never made it home with their parents, passing away in utero or shortly after entering the world.

When I did finally bring my son home after he spent two weeks in neonatal intensive care unit (NICU), it was these same women who I had spent time with in the hospital that I leaned on the most when I was having rough days. We used Facebook as our main way of sharing questions, concerns, and successes, since most of our babies were born preterm. While I had friends who had also recently given birth, their pregnancies were relatively uncomplicated and their stories of their babies sleeping through the night were something I couldn't relate to, and quite frankly, made me unfairly resent them.

As my son has grown and our list of treatments, medical appointments, and tests has increased, I continue to find it very valuable to connect with parents on a similar journey. This will also serve you well as these connections will play a critical role in supporting you as you advocate for your child. By sharing stories and experiences with other parents, you will be able to identify common obstacles, inconsistencies in support, as well as share resources that are available. Through these connections you will find new pieces to the puzzle and allow you to have a better understanding of the support, care, and services available for your child.

Through work I have been able to connect with a mother whose daughter has some similar challenges to my son. Living in a smaller community, we share the same pediatrician and have seen many of the same specialists. She is one of the few people I fully confide in. She has been a huge support in sharing stories, offering her perspective, and most importantly, reminding me that I'm not alone. We have also switched our children's pediatrician appointments, when one of us has a need to get in earlier to see her, but the doctor's calendar is full.

Through our friendship we are able to share our frustrations, our successes, things we've learned, and challenges we are facing. The benefit with our sharing is one of us is emotionally involved, as it is our child, while the other is listening as a parent who is familiar with the challenges and resources available. Often one of us is able to provide the other with clear advice from a parent who has been there, done that, or at least going through a similar journey. This connection and support has helped each of us in our role as advocates for our children. It has also helped us realize our struggles are not unique, and no, we aren't crazy in feeling the rollercoaster of emotions that goes with raising children, especially children with special needs.

Since my son is a couple of years older than her daughter, she's also able to learn tools to help her daughter as I share my process of advocating for my son to have an educational assistant at school and other challenges facing children as they grow. These conversations often involve me stopping mid-walk, turning to her and saying, "Take note of this. You'll want to remember this obstacle and how I tackled it when your daughter starts school." One parent's lesson learned is another parent's knowledge to help navigate a similar situation.

When I'm in the middle of a particular issue, I'm grateful to be able to have someone to talk things through with and get honest feedback from someone who truly understands and appreciates the challenges. This is particularly helpful in advocacy situations to know I'm not alone, my frustrations are real, and that I have the support I need to keep fighting. Our friendship and common obstacles motivates me to advocate versus giving up, as I know my advocacy will help remove or, at the very least, decrease some of the same obstacles her daughter, and other children, may also face.

While it can be tempting to cocoon your family and yourself away during challenging times, it's important you not only take stock of your support system, but also make an effort to connect with other parents in the quieter times so you have people to help you when you need them most. You can meet other parents at school, therapy sessions, through church, or through other parents or family members.

The point is to pull yourself up, take a look around you, and make these important connections with other parents. These connections aren't just about helping you, but you may also find you are able to play a key role in supporting another parent in his or her journey. At the end of the day, these connections will ultimately benefit your child, as you will have additional support and energy to tackle this important job of parenting.

See Exercise 5 (also available on the download kit) about asking for help.

Exercise 5
Asking for Help

Asking for help can be a difficult thing to do for many people. We are often limited by our thoughts that our problems are private, that we don't want to bother others, or that no one really understands what we are going through. But think back to times when people have asked you for help. Did you turn the person away or did you find ways that you could help in your own way? You likely looked at the situation and found a way to lend your support. This could include driving someone to an appointment, bringing over a meal, or just sitting and listening to his or her concerns.

The first step in asking for help is to get clear on what specific help you need. This allows people to help you in a meaningful way and provides direction to people who say, "Let me know if you need anything." Too often we thank them for the offer but don't follow up with a list of ways they can provide meaningful help.

This exercise is designed to help you get clear on what help you need and how your friends, family, neighbors, and coworkers can best support you and your family during the difficult times.

How long do you need support? Is it for a set period while your child is having a medical treatment or longer-term support?

Do you need help with meals?

What types of meals does your family enjoy?

If friends were to provide food, what is the best way of helping you in meal preparation? Example: Already prepared meals that just require heating or preportioned and chopped ingredients for a family member to put together. Be clear on what foods your family likes so you don't end up with a freezer full of tuna casserole no one will eat.

What support do you need inside of the home?

☐   Cleaning

☐   Laundry

☐   Meal preparation

☐   Visits

☐   Babysitting or play dates so you and/or your partner can take a break

☐   Babysitting or play dates while you take your child to medical appointments

☐   Other:

What support do you need for your children? Is there a specific date and time for these items or a regular day that is challenging?

Homework support

Play dates

Drop off/pick up of children from school/daycare

Getting your children on/off the bus

Shuttling your children to their extracurricular activities

Taking care of a child/children overnight while you are away with your other child for treatment

Other:

What support do you need outside of the home?
- [ ] Picking up groceries
- [ ] Other:

What friends/family/coworkers have offered support (the 'let me know if you need anything' statement)? Also include anyone you know who could offer support both locally and remotely. List all

What are your greatest stresses?

The next step is to review your answers above and fill out the following chart. The column on the left is support needed. In the top row fill in the names of friends and family members who can help, checking the appropriate support they can provide based on your relationship and comfort level. I've left room for you to enter other forms of support.

SUPPORT NEEDED						
Meal prep	☐	☐	☐	☐	☐	☐
Cleaning	☐	☐	☐	☐	☐	☐
Rides	☐	☐	☐	☐	☐	☐
Groceries	☐	☐	☐	☐	☐	☐
Laundry	☐	☐	☐	☐	☐	☐
Visits	☐	☐	☐	☐	☐	☐
Babysitting/ play dates	☐	☐	☐	☐	☐	☐
Picking up children	☐	☐	☐	☐	☐	☐

Having children overnight	☐	☐	☐	☐	☐	☐
	☐	☐	☐	☐	☐	☐
	☐	☐	☐	☐	☐	☐
	☐	☐	☐	☐	☐	☐
	☐	☐	☐	☐	☐	☐

This table will help you visualize how the people in your life can help you in a variety of ways. The final task is to ask for help in a clear and specific way. How you do this can vary on your relationships. You can send a mass email to all of your friends/family/coworkers using the template below or you can have individual conversations using this exercise as a tool on what you and your family's specific needs are and how they can offer support. What is important is that you are specific on the support your family needs and how each person can help.

Draft email

Hi family and friends,

I'm sorry for this group email, but I've found this is the best way to communicate and provide an update on our situation. *Insert why you are asking for help. Your child is booked for medical treatment or you're going through a rough patch. You don't need to give all the details, but let them know a bit about your situation and why you need help. Your friends and family likely already know a bit, but it's important to relate to them how this challenge is tied to your request for help.*

Some of you have offered your help to our family. Instead of putting anyone on the spot, I thought it would be best to send a group email letting you know the support our family needs during these challenging times.

In the home
Laundry
Cleaning

Meal preparation (either helping at meal time or supplying healthy prepared meals) *Be specific here on what you and your family like and don't like.*

For the children
Homework support
Play dates
Babysitting
Sleepovers

Outside the home
Picking up groceries
Dropping off/picking up our children from bus/school/daycare *Be specific on times/locations.*
Shuttling children to extracurricular activities *Be specific on times/locations.*

I'm hoping this list will help you better understand the support we need during this challenging time. My family and I are happy for any help you can give us.

I thank you for all your love and support.

Your name

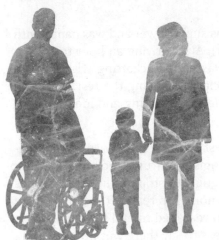

5

Dealing with Roadblocks

Dealing with roadblocks is an all too common challenge for caregivers of children with special needs. It can be even more difficult to navigate these roadblocks for families with children who have lesser-known needs, as they don't have the better-understood labels of autism or ADHD and the resources, support, and acceptance that go with these diagnoses.

Before you can work on removing the roadblocks, you first need to be clear on your child's strengths, his or her specific needs, the specific actions that are required and identify who can help remove these roadblocks. You know your child better than anyone else. While the medical system sometimes leans towards a cookie cutter approach, you know what will work for your child and what won't work. Don't ever forget that. It is one of your superpowers as your child's advocate. You know your child better than anyone, so listen to your gut and don't second guess your intuition. A wise family doctor once told me that early in his medical training he learned to listen closely to parents, as 90 percent of the time their instincts are right as they are better tuned into their child and his or her needs than anyone else.

As I mentioned earlier, after a year of endless medical appointments, my son discovered his superpower in medical situations was to not talk or cooperate, thereby taking back some of the control. He had realized his stubborn streak could work in his favor.

At one hearing test, he tested this superpower and was happy with how successful it was (to my despair). After driving an hour to the appointment, during which time he was happily chatting with me and singing to his music, he decided to clam up during the test. Not ideal when the test was to determine his level of hearing and identify what sounds he could and couldn't hear.

Instead of trying to make the test fun and get my son to participate, the person assisting the audiologist got frustrated and said, "Listen, if you're not going to speak, I'm going to stop playing these games with you." Now, my son was smart enough to realize the games were the test, so he was happy when she threatened to end the games, as it meant the test would be over. Needless to say there was no recovering from the comment and we left the hearing test without it being finished and driving the hour back home. It was a frustrating morning for everyone involved; except for my son who was pretty proud of himself for getting the upper hand on the assistant.

This outing reminded me why I need to take an active role in testing situations, setting the stage in advance for everyone involved, instead of sitting back passively while the experts take control. I knew my son best, and what would motivate him to participate, but hadn't been speaking up on his behalf, which had resulted in some challenging medical visits. With my son, I now clearly explain to him ahead of time not only what test he is having done, but also why it is important that he participate in the test.

Having rediscovered the role I needed to play in ensuring his voice was heard in assessments, after he had his drainage tubes placed in his ears, we had to return to the same clinic for another hearing test. Before we left the house I took the time to explain to my son that the hearing test was to let the doctor check if the tubes were working and draining the fluid in his ears that had made it hard for him to hear. I reminded him how we had gone to the hospital for the operation; how it had helped him to hear better and that we wanted to make sure the tubes were still in his ears and doing their job.

When we got to the clinic, I then took the audiologist aside, explained how my son has had numerous medical appointments and how he had learned he could be in control of these appointments by not participating. I also reminded her of the frustrating experience we had all had at the previous hearing test. Through this conversation she was able to see my child as a person, knowing in advance how he reacts to testing and adapting her test to meet his individual needs.

This time the hearing test began with the audiologist asking my son if he wanted to see his ears on the television or see the lines on a chart that reflected the sounds he was hearing. He picked the television. Starting the visit with a choice allowed him to maintain some control. She then made a point of showing him the drainage tubes in his ears, letting him see what color they are, and explained how they worked. We spent a few minutes looking at the tubes, which allowed him to further understand the recent operation and make the connection with what was now in his body and how it was helping him to hear.

The audiologist then told my son that the games in the hearing test booth were designed to make sure the tubes were doing their job and that he could hear all the different sounds. She acknowledged the games were part of the hearing test and why he needed to participate. She asked him if he would like to play the games so she could check on his hearing. She then allowed him to choose the games. Once again he had some control and was playing an active role in the test versus just being told what to do and expected to participate.

It was this subtle difference in approach that resulted in a successful hearing test and less frustration for everyone involved. This happened because I was clear on my son's needs, and advocated for the action required to have a successful test. While this might seem like an obvious process, it is these small advocacy moments that can clearly show us the benefits of advocating for our child. It also empowers us for the larger challenges. Most importantly, it demonstrates to your child that you are there to support him or her, and will be his or her voice.

I have shared this story with other parents, and they have often commented that while it seems so obvious and simple, the small advocacy moments are something they don't often practice. Instead they enter the test with their child, get frustrated when their child doesn't cooperate, grumble at yet another challenging experience, and leave feeling upset. By taking a step back and critically assessing your role and your child's needs, taking a proactive approach can result in a less stressful situation and more positive outcome for everyone involved. It is these small victories that can help prepare you and your child for the bigger challenges.

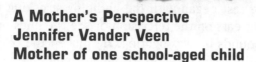

A Mother's Perspective
Jennifer Vander Veen
Mother of one school-aged child

The parent is the first advocate for a child. You as a parent know your child intimately, and you can sense when something is wrong, or doesn't feel right. You are the only advocate that is 100 percent invested in the well-being of your child, and you can keep a running tally in your head about when to advocate, and when to step back and trust an expert/doctor/other caregiver.

Your "gut" or subconscious is very good at processing information about your child at lightning speed. You will know before anyone else when your child is in trouble, is experiencing a life-threatening event, is in need of medical attention beyond that of a family doctor or non-specialized practitioner, or when your child is "off" in any way.

When your child is very young and unable to communicate, does not communicate well, or at all, then you are essentially an arm of his or her experience. You must speak up and be heard FOR your child, since he or she is incapable of expressing that need.

For a parent of a child with ANY special needs, the parent should never have to pick battles or be made to feel inadequate, fearful, inferior, uninformed, bullied, or feel as if he or she is just being a nervous parent. Any medical provider who sloughs you off, minimizes your concerns, doesn't seem invested or interested, and tries to fix the child, rather than accept, treat, and support the child, is not a good fit. You should not be at the mercy of a bad provider! While fighting for your child is noble, it shouldn't always feel like a battle.

Never ever feel sheepish, ashamed, or timid about getting second opinions, or various approaches to a problem. That is your prerogative!

That being said, I wouldn't suggest ticking off your child's medical team as you need to work together. Things that tick off a medical team include branching out of your scope and requesting irrational things that will not help your child. Pestering medical professionals is only necessary in a few situations.

Being unkind and eschewing their expert advice is a bad idea too, unless you feel like you are backed up with evidence to do so. Being seen as informed and assertive, rather than Mama Bear or Papa Bear, is much more efficient and helps you be taken more seriously by medical professionals.

Take space when medical professionals are rushed. Purposefully tell them that you require their time and why. When you can, have any issues, questions, concerns, or topics either recorded on video or written down for appointments. Wasting time is not received well by the medical profession.

Importance of Self-care

Advocating for your child can be exhausting. Because it places a burden on the parent, the parent must take strides to have good self-care or breaks to avoid caregiver burnout. Advocating can feel never ending and repetitive. It can feel lonely ... like you are the only one who really cares about your child's needs. You also may find you can never really relate to other parents who have children without special needs.

It is difficult to find a great team to help your child and find ways to relieve your anxiety. Sometimes it feels like you aren't doing enough, when you really are. Self-awareness, self-care, and self-forgiveness are great tools for the advocating parent. It is important to have a good social support network ready, and consider personal and family/couples therapy when YOU need to talk and feel supported. Don't feel ashamed of struggling with your own issues such as depression, burnout, mental health issues, fatigue, etc. Having a child [with] special needs is difficult in and of itself: being an advocate is a lot on top of that, and adds an additional level of stress.

Being the Expert

Advocating for your child is a part-time job. Unfortunately your child is a number to the outside world, and you need to be a squeaky wheel to be heard, even if that is not your personal style or natural inclination. However, you can still be kind, but firm when making your voice heard.

Remember, knowledge truly is power. This means knowing your enemy, and researching your child's syndrome, condition, illness, disabilities, and needs. Know your child's details almost as if it is your profession or special field. You may find that in some instances, you know more than a person working in a specific field, and that is OK.

Getting Support

Find people in your caregiving circles who take your word at face value and take you seriously. Take the time to determine if they actually care about your family and your child.

You'll know if someone cares about your child because you will feel a bond of trust, and you'll be relaxed with him or her and he or she will demonstrate that your child matters to him or her. Your child will feel relaxed with that person, too. If your hackles go up when speaking with a medical provider, and you are not being heard as a parent, then you need to pinpoint what it is that bothers you. It may mean it's time for you to consider shopping around for another provider (if that luxury is available to you).

To support you on this journey, you need to seek out other parents who have similar children to commiserate with, rejoice with, and share with. The more you know, the better advocate you will be, as you will be armed with tools to help you speak up for your child, or allow your child to speak up with assistance. You'll know what resources are available. You'll know when a prescribed treatment may or may not be recommended or warranted. You'll be aware of how to avoid pitfalls and being misled down other paths that can waste your time, money, energy, and resolve for certain treatments, programs, appointments, specialists, etc.

Family and friends are sometimes great allies, but they can also be great foes (usually inadvertently)! You may need to advocate more strongly and vocally with relatives if they minimize your child's needs, or do not take you seriously. You may need to explain and write up in detail the needs of your child so they are aware.

Sadly you may also need to cut some people out of your life, or to draw up strict boundaries. Only do this when there is a threat of harm to your child. Family and friends should be allies and fellow advocates, as the support of your village is very important to the health and wellness of your child.

Reaching Out

Don't be timid or afraid to reach out to all people involved in your child's care, and enlist help when needed. For example, make sure teachers, daycare providers, school bus drivers, school principals, doctors, nurses, therapists, and anyone highly involved in the life of your child know the ins and outs of your child's condition and needs.

Write it out, draw it out, say it out loud, and make copies! Then have specialists, occupational or physical therapists, other therapists, doctors, surgeons, etc., send letters detailing your child's condition and needs so you have third party credibility, and emergency contacts to get things done.

For example, my child requires an educational assistant (EA) in her classroom when she eats. I wrote the school principal, the classroom teacher, met with both, then had an occupational therapist and my daughter's surgeon detail her condition in writing. This effort resulted in our request for an EA being approved by the school board, ensuring my daughter is safe and an emergency protocol is in place should something happen.

A Success Story

My daughter was born with a birth defect (tracheo-esophageal fistual and esosphagea atresia), and an extra thumb. She needed her esophagus detached from her trachea and rebuilt so she could eat and breathe properly. She had her first surgery at four days old. The surgeon told us all of the potential complications of the surgery, and that we should look for those complications once we were back at home.

A week after being released from the neonatal intensive care unit, my daughter started vomiting after nursing for no apparent reason. It got worse, and at one time, I stayed awake all night so she could get enough to eat and be safe if she vomited. I definitely knew something was very wrong.

I recalled being told by the surgeon that she could develop a stricture; a narrowing of her esophagus. It was common, and since she was growing and had sutures and scar tissue in her esophagus, I wondered if she had one. I figured that meant going back to the hospital for a dilatation (a stretch) procedure to make her esophagus bigger again so she could get milk down.

I told my husband I thought we should go to the emergency room as my daughter was now vomiting profusely, getting dehydrated, and seemed to have very raspy breathing. He did not think that was necessary as we were already burned out from our last hospital stay, and I was suffering with the recent trauma and subsequent post traumatic stress (PTSD) symptoms of a violent birth and finding out that my daughter's life was threatened.

While I understood his concerns, I insisted that something was wrong. At the emergency department, two different pediatricians (who were aware of my daughter's medical history and surgery) completely dismissed my concerns. One told me I was just being a nervous new mom. The other said, "What are you so worried about? The X-ray is clear. Just go home and relax."

I felt completely unsettled leaving the hospital. I knew something wasn't right. I couldn't understand why I was rudely dismissed and sent home so quickly.

That night, I was up again all night, worried sick and crying while my daughter struggled to nurse, then vomited, followed by raspy breathing.

The next day, I called my aunt who is a nurse. I voiced my concerns and she came over right away. I told her the situation and she encouraged me to follow my gut. She drove me to my family doctor as I had booked a same-day appointment for my daughter.

The nurse practitioner could also not find anything wrong with my daughter. "Perhaps you are just being hyper-vigilant as a nervous, new mom?" she suggested. I left feeling defeated and angry. Clearly, something was abnormal. I had had enough.

In my exhaustion, worry, and very angry mind, I paged my daughter's surgeon directly. I described everything and she immediately said, "You need to come into emergency right away. Your daughter needs a dilatation procedure. You were right; and by the way, mom knows best."

I grieved and rejoiced simultaneously, then packed our hospital bags. My daughter had a test to confirm the diagnosis, and had the procedure the next morning.

I was jubilant in my mother's instincts and that I had researched what I could about my daughter's condition so I was prepared. I was also disappointed [in] and outraged [at] the people who dismissed me as being a nervous new mom.

At the end of the day I was thankful I had advocated for my daughter; had I not, she could have aspirated, suffered organ damage, or even died. Never again, would I bend my will and subject myself to another's scrutiny when the doubt was shouting at me from within.

1. Advocating versus Bullying

In speaking with my son's medical team as I was writing this book, one of his specialists asked that I include a piece about advocating versus bullying. She proceeded to tell me a cautionary story about a particularly aggressive mother she encountered in her practice.

This doctor told me she had referred one of her patients to a large teaching hospital a couple of hours away to be seen by a different specialist as the child's needs exceeded the care she could provide. The referral was made, and the doctor explained to the parents that the hospital would call them when an appointment was available. She also explained that due to the specialized support required and long waiting list, it would likely be a few months before the child would have an appointment.

A couple of weeks after the referral had been made, the mother called the office of the referring doctor, asking when would her son have an appointment. The doctor's receptionist explained the process for referrals, reminding the mother that it would be the hospital calling with the appointment information, not the referring doctor.

A week went by, and the mother called the referring doctor's office again, demanding to know the date of her son's appointment at the hospital. Once again, the receptionist explained the process. Not happy with the answer, the mother insisted on speaking to the specialist (who had her own extensive caseload). The specialist called the mother back, and explained the referral process for the third time.

The next day the mother called again, this time screaming at the receptionist, saying she didn't care if it was up to the hospital to call her. She wanted the referring specialist to get an appointment date for her son and that she would call back every day until her son had an appointment. She continued to call on a daily basis, insisting the referring doctor needed to take action to get her son an appointment.

In sharing this story with me, the specialist said she wanted caregivers to know there is a line between advocating and bullying. Advocating doesn't mean screaming, shouting, treating people disrespectfully, and insisting on the impossible. That is bullying and unfortunately, bullying only hurts the child, as doctors may avoid dealing with the family. After all, they are people too and want to avoid conflict.

In this child's case, the doctor who was being verbally abused was the only specialist in their area of expertise in the area, with the next closest being a ferry ride away. So while it may be frustrating to wait for a referral appointment, taking the frustration out on the medical office trying to help the child is not a good approach. Rather, a calm discussion with the receptionist or doctor about who to call at the hospital to discuss the delay would be more beneficial in helping the child getting the care he or she needs. This way the questions about the appointment would have been directed at the clinic that was booking the appointment.

The specialist who relayed this story said she would like caregivers to understand the role everyone plays in caring for a child. Caregivers need to be a productive team member versus an obstacle. Advocating is about understanding your child's needs, working with his or her medical team, and, when needed, pushing back in a respectful versus threatening manner. After all, you want your child's medical team to be positively involved in his or her case, not see you as the barrier.

2. Knowing Your Child's Rights

Your child is a person, not just a patient. His or her needs will depend on his or her age, mood, the time of day, and medical challenges. Regardless of these needs and his or her level of engagement, children have the right to be treated with respect, sensitivity, and dignity.

You also have rights as a parent. You have the right to make decisions on behalf of your child. Unless life threatening, you have the right to take your time, review information, and consult with your medical and personal support team before making a decision. You have the right to ask as many questions as you need in order to understand the situation. You have the right to advocate for your child without being seen as a problem or nuisance.

When my son was four years old, I had to remind the medical system of these rights — twice within a month. The first incident was when we had driven in a snowstorm for an MRI we had been waiting three months for my son to have. We had left our home early in the morning as we had learned the highway over the mountain was closed and we had to take a ferry to get to the hospital, which was in another city. Since our son was being sedated for the procedure, he wasn't allowed to have anything to eat or drink after midnight. So you can imagine what mood he was in for the hour-long car drive. Adding to the stress, the snowstorm had closed the schools, so our daughter was spending her snow day in the car with us not building snowmen, as she had hoped. We now had two unhappy passengers.

After a white-knuckle drive, we arrived at the hospital, checked in at admissions, and made our way to the pediatric unit. When we found the nurse she said, "Oh, you are here. I left you a message saying we are short staffed and the MRI likely won't happen today." I stood there with two unhappy children and a tired husband, with my mouth hanging open. When we had registered at the front desk mere minutes earlier they had confirmed all of our cell numbers, so I knew the hospital had our contact information.

I informed the nurse the highway over the mountain was closed and we had needed to leave our house early in the morning to catch the ferry. I asked why she didn't call our cell numbers, to which she responded she left us a message — at our home. She shrugged her shoulders and said, "Well you're here now, and we'll see what we can do."

Our son was assessed, put in a hospital gown and we were sent to a room to wait for his appointment. Five minutes before his scheduled MRI, the doctor came in to tell us the MRI was canceled as they had a medical emergency and no longer had a pediatric nurse to accompany our son. He then gave us a new date for the MRI, with this appointment being another two months away. By now it was 1:30 p.m., and our son hadn't had anything to eat or drink since 6:00 p.m. the night before. We took our cranky kids to the cafeteria to get food and then drove home. On the drive we had to explain to our son why he didn't have his picture taken (which is how we had explained the MRI) and that we would have to go through the entire process over again in a couple of months. He was not at all happy about this, and much of the ride home involved tears — from both kids.

To my credit I waited until the next day to call the patient office at the hospital to complain. I took the time to work through all of my various emotions and frustrations, and to gather my thoughts for the call. Instead of screaming at the person at the other end, I put on my patient advocacy hat and made some notes so I would stay focused. I knew from previous experiences that while crying and screaming may be therapeutic in the moment, it does little to advance your case and get your message across. After all, this was about my son getting the support he needed, not me ranting about my frustrations.

I explained to the patient complaint office that the hospital had put my family's safety at risk by not making an effort to contact us at all of our registered phone numbers to let us know the MRI would likely be canceled. Yes, we had ventured out in a snowstorm on our own accord, but we did so weighing the serious condition for which our son needed an MRI versus the road conditions as well as the long waitlist if we had rescheduled. I asked for clarification on the hospital's policies on contacting patients when there were anticipated changes to appointments. I learned the hospital's protocol was to call all available numbers a minimum of five times, leaving messages at each number, if necessary, for out-of-town patients. I asked to speak to someone who would be able to discuss my son's specific case, knowing the person in the patient complaint office was simply the frontline staff member and had little ability to do more than listen.

Later in the day the manager of the imaging department called me to discuss my concerns. She was very apologetic about our situation and confirmed the hospital's policy for calling all numbers on file was not followed in our son's situation. Wanting to advocate for not just my son but also other parents, I asked if she could meet with the manager of the pediatric unit to ensure the nurses there were aware of and followed this same policy on consistent basis. She had told me it had been a busy day on the pediatric floor, which is why only one phone call was made. I walked her through our family's journey to get to the hospital so she could relate to my frustration and the stress of the nurse doing the bare minimum had caused not only our son but also our entire family. A stress that could have been avoided by spending two more minutes trying to reach us on our cell phones.

It was by walking through our day that she finally understood what my true concern was and what resolution I was looking for to ensure this didn't happen to other families. I did my best to minimize the emotions and focus on the facts involved in out-of-town families getting to medical appointments that have long waitlists. I also explained that we were well aware of the reality that if we missed our MRI appointment our son would go to the bottom of the waitlist and it would take months to get a new appointment, which is another reason we ventured out in bad weather to get to the hospital.

After a rather productive conversation, the imaging manager was able to get our son an MRI appointment in a month's time. Instead of grumbling about how long of wait that was, I thanked her for the appointment and asked for a note to be made in our son's file that if there was any change we were to be called at all of our phone numbers on file. When the day came for the MRI there were no issues. Clearly that note had been made on our son's file as when we arrived at the hospital everyone assured us that our son would indeed have his MRI that day.

Sadly, less than a month later I was on the phone with the same patient complaint office. This time it was due to a phone call from our local hospital (that is part of the same health network). I was told my son's surgery for ear drainage tubes had been canceled, as the anesthesiologist wasn't available for a presurgery consult until Wednesday at 8:30 a.m. — the morning of his surgery. The kicker was I was getting this phone call at 11:00 a.m. on the Monday, less than 48 hours before his surgery.

Once again I put on my patient advocacy hat and asked whom I could speak to about this decision. Despite my annoyance, I knew the person calling me was the booking clerk and had no power to change the situation. This is something that is important to remember as you advocate for your child. You need to determine who is the messenger and who is the person who can take action. There is nothing to be gained by dumping your frustrations on the messenger. They may even put new roadblocks in your path if you treat them with disrespect. I've found if I treat them kindly and stress that I'm upset at the situation, not them, they actually find ways to help me. Sometimes it's as simple as connecting me with the person who can make a decision or someone who is in a role of authority.

The booking clerk then referred me to the manager of the operating room, but warned it was highly unlikely there would be any change to the surgery cancellation. So much so that the receptionist went ahead and rebooked his surgery for a future date. I asked her to give me three hours and hold his current appointment until I was able to make some phone calls. I told her a bit about my son's situation and the fact his hearing was severely impaired and the surgery was crucial in restoring his hearing. By giving her this insight, I hoped she would see my child as a person versus a name on a list. It worked as she agreed to hold on to the spot until 2:00 p.m.

I hung up the phone, went outside, got some fresh air, and then spent the next three hours making phone calls. As with the MRI situation I made sure I had given myself some time (in this case five minutes) to gather my thoughts instead of reacting with raw emotions.

My first call was to the ear, nose, and throat (ENT) office, letting them know the hospital had canceled the surgery (they were unaware), and that I had three hours to try and reverse this decision. I asked them to also hold the spot (in the event the hospital called), as I knew they had a waiting list for this valuable operating room time.

My next call was to the same patient complaint office as before. As luck would have it, I spoke to the same individual as my previous call. He was very apologetic that I had to call the office twice in a month about the same child. He told me the office's policy is to return calls within three to five business days, but due to the urgency of my situation he would speak to his manager immediately.

I explained my main concern with the canceled surgery was the emotional trauma it could cause my son. He had spent most of the weekend asking questions about IVs, the operation, the operating room, and the doctor. I explained that my son was not a typical child as he is in the medical system on a frequent basis. I also shared he had a bad association with this particular hospital, as the last time he was there he was having a seizure and he ended up spending a week in the hospital. Again I made an effort to provide insight on my child as a person, his fears, and needs, rather than focusing on my personal frustrations.

My third phone call was to leave a message for the manager of the operating room, who ultimately was responsible for establishing and monitoring the operating room schedule. After a nervous hour of waiting and watching the minutes tick away, she called me back. It was evident in our conversation that she had spoken with the manager of patient complaints, as she knew the background story. Even so, I repeated my concern about the potential for my son to have two procedures canceled with short notice, and the fact he would have to relive all the stress and anxiety he had in preparing for a future surgery date.

I had also learned, through a phone call with the ENT office, that the hospital admission clerk had overlooked the original referral for an anesthesiologist consult when the surgery was first booked. It was only when our family doctor submitted the preadmission paperwork that the requirement for an anesthesiologist was logged, which was on the Friday prior to the surgery. Through more questions, I learned that the requested anesthesiologist consult was only a five-minute appointment.

Armed with this information, I asked the operating room manager to find a way to have an anesthesiologist see our son before his Wednesday surgery, as the oversight on the consult was on the hospital's end.

After a few phone calls from the manager to the anesthesiologists, she was able to find an anesthesiologist who could meet my husband and son the afternoon before his surgery. This appointment lasted only a couple of minutes, with the anesthesiologist taking a quick history and examining our son — in the lobby of the hospital between his other appointments. As the assessment ended, the anesthesiologist told my husband he didn't know why his wife (me) had to be so difficult, and what was the big deal with the surgery being delayed a few weeks. When my husband relayed this message to me, I chose to let this comment go.

On the Wednesday morning my son went to the hospital for his surgery and was admitted without any challenges. While he was in the recovery room, the ENT doctor came out to talk to my husband and me. He told us he was glad our son had had the surgery, as the fluid in his ears was so thick his ears were essentially glued shut and his hearing would have been severely impaired. He explained the fluid would not have been able to drain on its own, and surgery was the only solution to restoring his hearing.

I thanked him and went outside to get some fresh air. While pacing outside I bumped into our family doctor and told him the story of the canceled surgery, my three hours of phone calls, and the comments from the ENT about the state of our son's ears. Our doctor shook his head and apologized for everything I had been through and acknowledged that it must have been a stressful three days for all of us. He told me I was 100 percent in the right and he was glad I had advocated for my son, as many parents wouldn't have gone through all the steps required to have a successful resolution. He told me how important it was that I continue to advocate, as each piece of advocacy work helps educate the medical system on the needs of patients, particularly children. While he wished advocacy wasn't needed, his hope was the cumulative effect of patient advocacy would slowly change the system.

This is why I share these two stories with you. Not so you can think, "Wow, she's quite a mama bear," but rather so you will see that by being an advocate for your child you are also advocating for other children. Hopefully through our collective advocacy we can make a difference.

As a footnote on this story, a year after my son's surgery I joined our district's health network as a patient advocate. One of the people who interviewed me for this volunteer position was the manager of the operating room to whom I had spoken when my son's surgery was originally canceled. She remembered our conversation and how calm, respectful yet assertive I had been. I hadn't become another barrier or been labeled as a difficult parent. In our interview she commented on how she wished more patients would take an active role in advocating in a respectful way.

Looking back on the conversation, the outcome, and the fact I now volunteer on a committee with this same doctor, it is a good reminder that in many communities, large and small, the healthcare team is interconnected. You never know when you may encounter a medical provider, so it's important to minimize the drama and find ways to discuss challenges in a way that allows you to work with them productively in the future, in the event your paths cross again.

3. Children's Needs versus Adult Needs

In both the situations covered in the last two sections, I spent time educating the doctors, nurses, and patient complaint staff (anyone who would listen) about the importance of and need to treat children differently from adults. I am continually concerned with how the medical system has one-size-fits-no-one approach to patient care.

I spent time explaining to the medical staff that a four-year-old child receives and processes information much differently than an adult. Canceling a surgery with two days' notice can be frustrating for adults, but it is a decision they can understand. They are able to process the information, appreciate the rationale behind the decision, ask appropriate questions, and move on. However, for children, a canceled procedure or surgery can be a traumatic experience. Preparing a child for surgery is much different than preparing an adult, particularly for children who already have negative associations with hospitals and doctors.

Most caregivers know the importance of helping children understand what will be happening to them. After all, it is their bodies and they need to be aware of what procedures will be done to them and by whom. In my son's case, he has had a few traumatizing experiences with IVs with medical staff taking up to one hour trying to get an IV into his body as his veins collapse easily. Because of this negative experience, he associates hospitals with IVs and IVs with pain; and for his surgery he knew he would need an IV.

As mentioned earlier, I spent the weekend answering a barrage of questions from my son about IVs, the surgery, and the operating room. While some of you might be thinking, why didn't I just wait until the day before the surgery to tell him, I know how my son processes information and last-minute conversations and surprise procedures do not end well. We watched YouTube videos, found pictures of ear drainage tubes, and talked about how the surgery would not only help him hear better but also allow him to hear new noises.

In my conversations with the medical team about the importance of understanding the needs of children versus adults, I walked them through how a child prepares for a procedure versus how an adult prepares. It was this personalization that helped get my message across and resonated with the medical staff.

It was never about the surgery or MRI being canceled and having to wait another few weeks. It was about a child getting emotionally and mentally prepared, and scared, about a procedure, it being canceled, and then having to go through the experience all over again. I explained how crucial it is for everyone involved to limit the stress on children by ensuring they have as limited contact with the medical system as possible and for each interaction to be as positive, or with as minimal trauma as possible.

Happy ending to this story: As I was putting my son to bed after his surgery I whispered to him, "I love you." He turned and looked at me with a huge smile on his face, and told me he heard me. He had never heard whispering before. I then whistled, a sound he had also never been able to hear, and he heard that too. The sheer joy on his face and the big hug he gave me as he experienced new sounds made all the stress, phone calls, and frustrations of keeping his surgery date worth it.

It's these small moments of joy that keep me motivated in advocating for my son. They are also good reminders that advocacy work can make a real difference to a child's health and well-being.

4. Accessing Support

The final message I want to share from my son's canceled procedures is to stress the importance of accessing all the support available in advocating for your child. Remember what I said at the beginning of this book: Patient advocacy isn't an individual but rather a team sport.

Pull on as many members of your team as possible and critically look at each situation to see who you can access to support your case.

Each situation is different. Sometimes your family doctor and pediatrician are enough. Other times you may need to include other medical specialists, therapists, and teachers. In extremely challenging situations you may need to expand your circle to include elected officials, ministry staff, hospital executives, and child advocacy organizations.

You also need to know when to pick your battles and determine what hills you are willing to die on. For me a canceled surgery with two days' notice was a battle I was ready to take on. I let snide comments slide, instead focusing my energy on the end result: getting an anesthesiologist's consult so my son's surgery would proceed. I also remembered this was never about my personal feelings, but about getting the best outcome for my son. He was the patient and I was his voice.

There are other times when I don't have the energy or willpower to take on the system. I know I should be advocating for my child, but frankly I know I am not up to the task. And that is OK too. I'm also aware of the careful balance between being seen as a complainer and being seen as a team member and concerned parent. I save my strength for the bigger issues that have a significant impact on his health and well-being. My battle to have an education assistant is another example of a battle I was prepared to take on.

As mentioned earlier in this chapter, it is important you are clear on your child, his or her needs and priorities for care. By fully understanding your child's bigger picture you will know when to put on your patient advocacy hat and fight for your child and when to trust in the medical system and its processes.

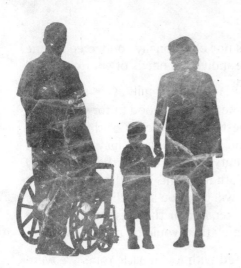

6
Find the Right Therapy for Your Child

Therapy plays an important role in helping children overcome, manage, or mitigate medical conditions or challenges. The list of therapy available is extensive, varying on your child's specific challenges as well as his or her personality, likes, and dislikes.

The first step in deciding on the right therapy for your child is a discussion with his or her case manager. While the case manager may not have all the answers, he or she can set the perimeters for your child and/or refer you to specific therapists for more insight. It is important you have clarity on your child's parameters up front and share this information. What are the no-go activities? What activities should be avoided as they can be dangerous for your child? What activities are ok, but in a modified form? What activities can your child participate in with little challenges? Children with coordination or mobility issues may not do well in team sports involving physical contact, such as hockey, soccer, or baseball. While this may seem obvious, too often I've seen parents project their own desires or aspirations on their children, without really listening and understanding what their child truly wants or needs. By discussing your child's condition, limitations, and recommended therapy with his or her case manager, you will have insights from a professional who is not emotionally connected to one activity, but rather is looking at the individual needs of your child and matching the activity to these needs.

Also, while you try and determine what is a good fit for your child, find out the type of therapy that best suits the needs of children with similar conditions. While your child's case manager may have some suggestions, this is a good opportunity to reach out to the community we discussed in Chapter 4 and ask other parents what has and has not worked well for their children. This will give you a baseline of activities to discuss with your child, caseworker, and/or therapist to determine which activities your child would enjoy that would be most beneficial.

When our son was first diagnosed with low muscle tone, we were referred to a physical therapist for an assessment. However, the wait to see her was about six months. In the meantime we had enrolled our son in swimming lessons, as they were held at the same time as our daughter's lessons, which was a motivating factor for signing him up for his own lessons. After a few sessions in the beginner group, the swimming instructor took us aside and told us our son would do better in private lessons as he wasn't progressing in the group setting, needed one-on-one attention, and was much bigger than the other kids in the class.

We found a mature swimming instructor (someone closer to my age versus a teenager) who understood how to work with our son and spent time slowly helping him overcome his fear of putting his face in the water. He didn't have to worry about keeping up with the rest of the class and he received the personal support he needed. He went from spending most of the class sitting on the steps of the pool, to enjoying going swimming and fully participating in his lessons. After three months of private lessons, our son made his way through all the beginner programs and was able to join a group lesson with children his own age. Not only did his skills advance but so did his comfort with being in the water. He went from resisting going into the pool to looking forward to our weekly outings. The one-on-one support truly made a world of difference in helping him progress and enjoy being in the water.

Towards the end of his private lessons, he finally had his physical therapy assessment, which looked at his fine motor and gross motor skills. While as parents we thought he had made huge progress and was doing great, which he had when tested on his individual progress not compared to his peers, the assessment found he was significantly behind his peers in his physical movements and development. This was a big blow as we were honestly not aware of how behind he really was, despite all of the work we had done with him.

After I had taken some time to have a good cry, I set up an appointment with the physical therapist to get her thoughts not only on his current needs, but also how to best support him as he grows. By asking for a set amount of time to review his assessment, we were both able to fully focus on the report and next steps. I highly recommend when you receive reports you don't just read the report, get frustrated, angry or cry, but rather set up an appointment with the appropriate therapist to review the report. Ideally this appointment should be at least a week after you receive the report so you have time to process the emotions so you are able to spend your time in the meeting dealing with the findings of the report on a factual versus emotional level. Too often when we go into these meetings with our emotions running high, we are not able to process all of the information and can miss out one hearing key points related to our child's treatment or care. Like other lessons I've shared in the book, this is also one I learned the hard way. I have since tried to break up my reaction to information. First, giving myself space and permission to react on an emotional level. Next sitting down and reviewing the report a few days later with a pen and paper, writing out any questions or comments. Then finally setting up a time with the medical practitioner or therapist to review the report or assessment, have my questions answered and, where appropriate, discuss next steps. Yes, it might seem like a bit of a process, but this way I'm able to focus on the information that's being conveyed without being a crying or screaming mess.

When it came to my meeting with the physical therapist to review my son's assessment, one piece of advice she gave me was to make sure I don't over-program him with activities (always a challenge for a Type-A mom) and to avoid running him from school to after-school activities. With his low muscle tone, he tires easily, and just going to school is enough activity for the day. This limited programming not only gives him time to rest, but also helps limit the amount of burnout for the entire family. As parents of a child with needs we already are managing doing speech therapy at home, as well as helping him work through episodes where his physical exhaustion appears as temper tantrums. It's actually freeing to know we have no activities after school, and can focus on making supper and spending time with our kids. This advice has also changed our daughter's extracurricular activities, so we don't have to drag our son with us from activity to activity, which would be just as exhausting for him as participating in his own activities. Instead, we keep our son's riding and swimming lessons to weekends, limiting each activity to one per day. The lessons are also in the morning, when he has the most energy and ability to concentrate. As for his sister, we have found a barn near our house where she can ride, limiting the amount of driving for us. Most of her lessons are also on the weekend. This doesn't mean we have stress-free nights, but it has helped eliminate the stress of running kids from activity to activity after working a full day.

Ultimately, you will need to discover what works for you and your family. Make sure when deciding what activities your child participates in you do so having a discussion with the case manager on what activities to avoid, limitations to participation, as well as limitations in how much activity (school and extracurricular) your child can handle in a day. See Exercise 6 (also available on the download kit).

1. Family Connection

I was fortunate that my daughter had fallen in love with horses and was riding weekly when we learned about the therapeutic horse-riding program that was available for our son. At first it was tough to realize that he would need therapeutic riding versus the same lessons as our daughter. I had to remember the point of the riding was to strengthen his core muscles, and he needed to be in a safe and supportive environment that best suited his needs.

Having spent hours at the horse barn watching his sister ride, I took the opportunity while at his sister's horse lesson to talk to my son about his interest in riding. Knowing he is a child who is hesitant to start new activities, I talked about how he could ride his own horse but that there would be people walking next to him to ensure he was safe. We watched some YouTube videos of children taking part in therapeutic riding. We then took him to the local therapeutic riding barn so he could meet the horses as well as the volunteers. This allowed him to gradually get used to the idea and be comfortable with the barn instead of just showing up one day for lessons without the transition period.

The first couple of lessons he wasn't sure about being on such a large animal since he had only been on a horse once before — and it was pony ride at the local fall fair. However, after a few months of riding lessons, I began to see not only his confidence building, but also his

Exercise 6
Finding a Therapy Fit for Your Child

When determining the appropriate therapy for your child, don't just look at what is available and force your child into a program or time that is not a good fit for his/her interests or energy levels. Rather, look at the bigger picture to determine your child's current needs, future needs, interests, and abilities, in an effort to find activities or programs that will best support him or her.

Here are some questions to help you select a program that best suits your child's needs, personality, and interests.

Questions for your child's case manager and/or therapist(s)

- What therapy would my child benefit from?
- How or will this change as my child develops?
- How should this therapy be delivered? One on one or in a group?
- Where can I access the therapy?
- What activities should my child avoid? Why (so you fully understand the reason for the restrictions)?
- What sports/activities can my child participate in? Group sports? Individual?
- What sports/activities should my child avoid?
- What information should I share with my child's coach/instructor to ensure his or her safety as well as to help him or her be successful?
- Are you aware of any financial support available for therapy? Either publicly funded or government/private/nonprofit support?

Questions regarding your child

- What interests him or her (any particular sports, activities)?
- Is there anything your child doesn't like (loud noises, crowds, getting wet)?
- Does he or she enjoy watching or being involved in any of his or her sibling's activities?
- What time of the day does he or she have the highest energy level and ability to concentrate?
- What time of day should be avoided?
- What activities are your other children involved in?
- What activities/sports are available in your community for children with similar needs?

Taking the time to answer these questions will give you a better idea of your child's needs, abilities, and interests. After you have completed this exercise, take time to discuss your findings with your child. Have a conversation with your child about which activities he or she enjoys. Depending on age, your child can sit with you filling out this exercise, looking at activities on the computer, and being involved in the decision-making process.

It can be tough for some caregivers to realize a child won't be playing competitive hockey or running track and field. What is important is setting up your child to be successful, which means finding activities and therapies he or she will enjoy.

ability to sit up straight and be in command of his horse. He went from whispering commands to his horse to saying them in a loud, confident voice. The change was amazing; as was the bond he had developed with his horse.

If it hadn't had been for our daughter's interest in horses, and conversations with her riding coach, I never would have known there was a therapeutic riding program in our community, or about the benefits it could provide to my son. I had been so focused on traditional physical therapy, not realizing that other sports and activities can also have therapeutic values.

I have also had to be honest about my son's needs. When we were first told he'd benefit from private swimming lessons, I was hurt. Spending every day with him, I didn't think he was different from his peers. The swimming instructor was very kind in how she explained his physical and developmental challenges, and how it would be better for everyone if he received one-on-one instructions.

I could have easily said no, he was fine in a group class, insisting he would catch up. Instead I decided to take her advice and see how he progressed in private lessons. Once he received his instructor's full attention, it was obvious how much he had been lagging behind in his group lessons. Even with having private lessons, it took two months before he'd put his face in the water and blow bubbles (even then infrequently and reluctantly). However, over time he was able to develop a relationship with his instructor, who soon learned how to motivate him. Most importantly, the instructor knew how to make his time in the pool fun. Now he loves going swimming and looks forward to his weekly trips to the pool with his educational assistant, as part of his school's swimming program.

For our son, all therapy and activities need to be fun. He has spent way too much time in medical settings, and as I mentioned earlier, tends to retreat when he's pushed to participate. Many kids with medical conditions are the same way. This is why it's so important to find activities they will enjoy, and to continue to make them fun. Otherwise, once the fun stops, so will their participation. They will cease getting the therapy they need, and you will be left struggling to find new activities.

So what does this chapter have to do with advocacy? Therapy is a huge part of every child's growth and development. For some it is done through sports. For others, through activities directed to meet their specific needs.

What is important is that you ensure your child doesn't get slotted into a program or activity he or she won't enjoy. Make sure you set your child up for success, not failure. Sure, it may be more convenient for the therapist to put your child in a group session, but is this something your child will enjoy? Will it motivate him or her to come back, week after week? Or will he or she resent the therapy while you spend most of the session trying to convince your child to participate?

It's important you don't just take what is offered in fear of offending anyone. Instead, dig deeper and truly understand your child's needs, interests, and abilities. This involves open conversations with your child about his or her likes and dislikes. If your child is too young to have these conversations, you can try out different activities and see which ones he or she gravitates towards and likes. Remember, with all kids it takes a few sessions before they fully understand the activity and are able to participate. Don't give up after one challenging session, but rather give yourself a set amount of time. For example, sign up your child for one session of swimming lessons. By the end of the lessons you will know if this is something your child loves, hates, or tolerates. Sometimes tolerates is the best you will get.

As you choose activities for your child, involve your child's case manager in the discussion. Before I enrolled my son in horse riding, I met with his pediatrician to get her thoughts on the benefits and risks of the program, how it would address his specific needs as well as have her fill out a doctor's referral for the program. She agreed with his physical therapist's endorsement, promoting the benefits of the program for building his core strength. She also gave me some parameters for his involvement and advice for his riding coach on his limitations. This information helped everyone involved, including my husband and I as we watched from the sidelines. We could all ensure he entered the program slowly, wasn't overtaxed, and most importantly, was riding in a setting that ensured his safety.

Once you have found a sport, a therapy, or an activity your child enjoys, make sure you remember to continually check back with your child's case manager as well as his or her therapist/coach, sharing any changes in your child's condition. One activity that may not have been allowed at year one may be acceptable in year three, or the other way around. Continue to check in with your child to see how he or she is enjoying the activity. Look for clues of when he or she needs a break, it's time to find a new coach, or your child has outgrown the activity.

Raising a child with special needs can be challenging and exhausting. Add taking on the role of patient advocate, and there are likely days when you wish you could close the curtains and sleep all day. During those times, what's most important is you focus on the immediate needs of you, your child, and your family. Taking the time to have some self-care, even if it just means shutting your bedroom door and picking up the phone to talk to a friend.

When you have some time to catch your breath, it is a good idea to set aside some time to reflect on your child's situation, the role you've played as his or her advocate and what is yet to come. This can be a quarterly or yearly reflection. What is important is you set aside time to review your situation and critically analyze your role as a patient advocate.

This isn't about beating yourself up and thinking I should have done this differently or I didn't advocate in that situation. Rather it is about trying to remove emotions from the review and reflect in an impartial manner (as much as can be expected when it comes to being a caregiver). See Exercise 7 (also included on the download kit).

Exercise 7
Annual Review

I would recommend setting aside a few hours to either sit with your partner or find a quiet space to work through this exercise by yourself. Give yourself the time and space to reflect on your patient advocacy achievements and setbacks over the last year. Spending the time to critically review your advocacy will help you identify successes, setbacks, and gaps to help you improve your advocacy skills. Remember, being an advocate for your child can be a lifelong journey, so it is important you take the time to review the past so you can improve in the future.

Here are some questions to help you conduct your personal review:

- Looking back on the last year, what are some of the personal successes your child has had? (This should be about your child, not his or her treatment/therapy, but rather your child as an individual. For some it's speaking more clearly, for others it's being able to climb independently.)
- What are some of the setbacks your child has faced?
- What therapy/activities is your child participating in?
- What is working?
- What is not working?
- What therapy/activities does he or she enjoy the most?
- What does he or she enjoy the least?
- In the last year, list all the times you advocated for your child. Be as specific as possible.
- Referring back to this list, what worked?
- What didn't work?
- Are there any common themes that have emerged? Example: Continually advocating for your child to have assessments in a timely manner. Or having to advocate for support for your child in a school setting?
- Reflecting on your patient advocacy, is there anything you would have done differently?
- Are there any lessons learned?
- Looking forward to the next year, are there any goals you would like to set for your patient advocacy?
- Where do you think you need to focus your patient advocacy energy?
- What areas do you think you can work on less?
- If you are doing this exercise a year from now, what do you hope to have achieved?
- What does success look like for you?
- What does success look like for your child?
- What support do you need to be successful? (Examples: training, counseling, better networking with other parents)
- What support does your child need to be successful?
- How can you recharge your batteries so you have the energy to advocate?

Once you have completed this exercise, you may want to make notes on anything that arises from this exercise that you want to discuss with your child's case manager and/or your support system. This exercise is inward facing, helping you get clear on your role as your child's advocate. Make sure you take the time to celebrate your successes and acknowledge all the hard work you've done to advocate for your child.

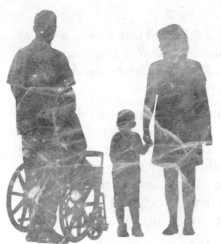

7
Share Your Story

We've all heard the saying "it takes a village to raise a child." As a parent you need to access and rely on your village during the good times and the challenging times. While it may seem easier to retreat from your village and cocoon your family at home as you struggle to deal with a challenge, this is the time you need to not only lean on your existing support system, but also work on expanding your circle to include other families or individuals who are on similar journeys.

I know firsthand how isolating it can be raising a child with special needs. It can be depressing to talk to friends with children the same age, and hear how their child has met milestones that my son is nowhere close to meeting. Or to listen to their child talking a mile a minute, and carry on a full conversation when my son's vocabulary still consisted of 100 words. While I try to remember that all children are different, and develop at their own pace, sometimes the stark reality of the large gap in development can be frustrating, depressing, and isolating.

Although I have tried over the years to confide in these friends about my fears and struggles, more often than not I've found they are either uncomfortable with the conversation or offer the blanket statement of, "It's OK. He'll catch up. You should stop worrying." I know they mean well, but unless you are raising a child with special needs or a medical condition, your friends and family cannot truly understand the everyday challenges, struggles, and small successes that come with raising these children.

It has taken me awhile, but I've finally discovered that my best support comes from friendships I've made with parents of children who also have special needs or medical conditions. In some cases, their children have some of the same conditions as my son. In other relationships their situation is much different or their children are now grown. What we do have in common is the variety of therapists and doctors to juggle, as well as similar challenges in navigating the system and getting support for our children.

It is the commonalities along our journeys as parents that have brought us together rather than our similarities as individuals. As you look to expand your support system, it is important you remember this difference so you don't miss out on making connections with people who can help you and your family. You will often have much different connections with these parents than you have with your existing friendships. These individuals will also play a much different role in your life. Sometimes they are people you might normally not be friends with due to differences in age, personalities, and geography. However, what will bring you together will be your passion and commitment to helping your children navigate similar obstacles.

Once I understood and accepted this difference, I found I was better able to open up to and be honest about my feelings with these new members of my support system. I know they won't judge me or tell me everything will be fine. Rather they are living through the same emotions, have encountered similar challenges, and can listen to my struggles from a true place of understanding that, as much as they may want to help, many of my other friends are not able to. I cannot tell you how valuable this subtle difference in friendship is in helping me get through the difficult times, or discussing everyday challenges and successes.

So how do you find these parents or individuals? Depending on your child's condition or challenges, as well as the community where you live, there may be a parent support group you can join. If these groups are available, seek them and make the time to connect and join one. Even if you can't attend every meeting, you will likely make some good connections and realize you aren't alone.

In my case, I have found these individuals in everyday situations, just by being open about my son and our journey. At first it was a struggle, as I wanted to keep our challenges private, especially since I wasn't working in a supportive work environment. I had actually been told that I was to keep my personal situation and struggles to myself, and not to share this information with work colleagues as it made some people uncomfortable.

While I tried for a few months to follow this "rule" I found it was making me feel more isolated and alone on my journey. I finally realized that by sharing my story with a few individuals I trusted, it would help them understand why I was absent for a few days and gave me someone to talk to on the rough days.

I made some great connections with some other moms at work. In a couple of cases they noticed I was absent from work for a week, and asked if I had been at home sick. When I opened up and explained I had been in the hospital with my son after a complex seizure, they also opened up about their children's medical conditions. One of these women was the mom I had mentioned earlier, whose daughter shares many of the same specialists as my son. It was our initial conversation following my son's hospitalization that resulted in us discovering our commonalities, which was a great relief to both of us knowing we weren't alone in our struggles. From this first conversation, we have become each other's main confidants. If one of us is having a rough day, we will go for a quick walk. Some days it is to offer advice. Other days it is just to have someone to listen to our concerns without judging.

We have found just having someone to talk to who truly understands our challenges, can be very therapeutic. It doesn't always mean they will have all the answers or offer sage advice that will solve a problem. But having the ear of someone who is on a similar journey helps me realize that I'm not overreacting and the emotions I'm feeling are valid, and often shared by her. We also share the small successes that only a parent on the same path would appreciate as milestone moments (such as her kid climbing up on a chair unsupported or being able to sit on the swing).

1. Community of Support

As you begin to reach out and form relationships with other caregivers, therapists, and medical staff, you will slowly find yourself part of a larger community. By developing personal and/or professional relationships with the members of your community, you will have their strength and support to draw on when you need to advocate for your child. Trust me, this is a much better place to be than fighting your battles on your own.

Remember, this is a two-way street. It's not just about getting people to support you. It's also about making meaningful connections and expanding your community by helping others.

I have become very open about sharing my struggles, successes, and lessons learned with other parents, therapists, and medical staff about my son's challenges as well as the advocacy work I've done on his behalf along the way. While this can be a vulnerable place to be as it lets people see behind the tough mask, it can also be very rewarding to know by sharing my experiences I'm helping either prevent a similar incident for another child or I am giving caregivers the confidence to know they too can advocate for their children.

How you share your challenges, successes, and ongoing struggles is up to you. It could be through creating or joining a social media group, and posting about your experiences. Some parents find blogging thera-peutic and a way of reaching a broader community. For others it can be through attending a support meeting, organizing a get-together with other caregivers, or through one-on-one conversations with friends. It can also be through formal meetings or informal discussions with members of your medical support team.

The important thing is to not keep this information to yourself, but rather find a way to share what you are going through with members of your community. Not only will it help you feel you aren't alone, but it may also result in more support for your child as others may have good advice or insight, or important connections to help you access the support needed.

If you are looking for a real life example of how a community can result in change, look at the support and therapy individuals with au-tism receive today versus 30 years ago. Sure, waiting lists for assess-ments and treatment can be long, but there are substantially more re-sources available and a better understanding of the condition.

How did this come to be? Part of the change has been the result of more children being diagnosed. Another main reason has been the strong advocacy work of parents over the years. As the autism commu-nity grew, the voices advocating for change became louder and more united. It is through this unity that both caregivers and medical providers were able to work together to get the resources needed to support children diagnosed with autism. This is a movement that continues to grow and offers great support for caregivers of children.

For some caregivers reading this book, your children have conditions that are not common or well understood. In other cases, your children have a variety of conditions and/or needs that individually are understood, but there is little appreciation for the support needed to address these collective challenges.

Regardless of which group your child belongs to, it is important that caregivers of these children, often the ones who fall through the cracks, find ways to seek others going through a similar journey. Often, by meeting the parent of a child with a similar condition, it will open the door to meeting more parents, learning about additional resources, and ultimately helping you better understand the support your child needs and how best to access this support.

You will also have a group of people to lean on during the difficult times. This may get you a sympathetic ear or the perspective of someone who is able to take a step back from the situation and accompanying emotions and offer a new approach or ideas on how to advocate for your child. You will have a community to reach out to and see if anyone has encountered a similar obstacle or challenge, how they dealt with it, and hopefully get insights on how to advocate for your child.

While it can be human nature to think you are the only person who has ever experienced a certain situation while you're going through a difficult time, you are likely not the first person to have had this struggle. Don't isolate yourself during these times, or you will truly be alone. Rather, realize this is when you need to reach out, clearly state the challenge your child is going through, and ask for the help, insight, or advice you need. You will be amazed how your community can help you and your family.

Also look for the common challenges your children are facing. Are there other children with your child's condition who also need a type of support that isn't readily available, or an alternative therapy? Are other caregivers struggling with similar issues, whether emotionally, financially, or by accessing resources? As the autism community has done raising awareness and advocating for treatment needed to support children, true change will only be made when caregivers and medical providers work together and have a united voice.

In my discussions with other parents I have also learned about a variety of resources and support available to my son and my family that I otherwise would not have known about. This includes government-funded speech, physical, and occupational therapies as well as community resources. Often, medical providers are overwhelmed dealing with the issues in front of them, and are not always aware of the various government funding, nonprofit funding, and programs available to caregivers and children. For this reason, it is important us caregivers share our knowledge with others versus keeping it to ourselves.

When I discovered how much therapeutic horse riding helped my son with his low muscle tone, I made sure I not only told other parents, but also shared my thoughts with all the members of his medical team. I did this so they would have a better understanding of therapeutic riding, its benefits, how to refer children to the program as well as financial support available for low-income families. My hope was by sharing what I had learned they too could share this information with other caregivers of children with low muscle tone. I had stumbled on a local program by accident, and wanted to help spread awareness so other caregivers would know about this program. At these riding lessons, I have also made great connections with other parents who have provided me insights on other programs and services my son can access. Joining one community can open up access to a whole other community.

I have also been vocal in sharing my advocacy success stories. Not only am I proud of the work I've done to get the support my son needs, but I also don't want other caregivers to go through the same stress and often unnecessary roadblocks. There are always lessons learned through advocacy work. Don't keep these to yourself. Share them. Share them with your friends, family, and community. Tell them what worked, what didn't, what you would do differently, and most importantly how it helped your child.

Also make sure you share these stories with your medical support team, especially your case manager. After my struggle with my son's canceled MRI and almost canceled surgery, I made a point of letting my son's pediatrician and family doctor know exactly what had happened, how I had dealt with it, and what changes I thought needed to be made to prevent this from happening to other children. In many communities, medical providers know each other, work at the local hospitals, and are able to advocate for change within the system versus outside the system.

It is important they understand the human element, how decisions impact children as people versus patients, and why change is needed. You don't want your medical team to just lend a sympathetic ear, but rather take the opportunity when telling your story to ask them to advocate for change on the inside, so either a situation isn't repeated or other children get similar support. They are important allies, and valuable members of the team in helping change the system to truly help children.

A Mother's Perspective
Caroll Taiji
Mother of six grown children

When my husband and I were going through the diagnosis, treatment, and associated medical challenges with our son more than 20 years ago, we didn't really understand how to effectively advocate on his behalf. In the early days we took our son to numerous specialists, trying to figure out what was going on with him. The panic of trying to get him the help he needed meant we did not always ask all the right questions.

As we got older and had a better understanding of the challenges facing our son, we became a little calmer and more surefooted about asking questions and doing the research.

Twenty years later, looking back on first few years of our journey, my advice to other parents is to be easy on yourselves. There isn't a more challenging and emotionally complex situation than worrying about a child who has medical challenges. It can be overwhelming and years later, it can still feel quite raw and emotional. But, the last thing you need to do is judge yourself. We are all doing the best we can under difficult circumstances and adding guilt and self-criticism to the fear and uncertainty is to be avoided if at all possible!

The hardest part is these feelings of concern and worry never truly go away. Know that you are not alone in what you are feeling. Reach out and share your experience with another parent on a similar journey so you can support each other.

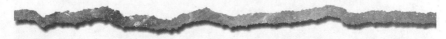

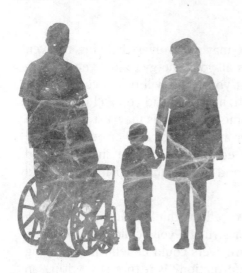

8
Giving Back

As you journey along the road of patient advocacy, you will find there are times when people in your support team are reaching out and helping you, and there are times when you are helping others. As you advocate for your child, you will have successes, encounter roadblocks, and have experiences that you will share with others.

Regardless of whether you have a positive or negative experience, what is important is that you share your experience with others. The first thing I mentioned in this book was the fact that patient advocacy is not an individual pursuit but rather a team sport, with all of your medical and support team having a role to play. The size of the role and their level of involvement will depend on the situation.

Part of your role is to pay forward the help you've received in order to help other caregivers and children. The knowledge you have gained, and will continue to gain on this journey could help another caregiver avoid or overcome similar obstacles.

How you give back depends on your situation. For some, it may just be reaching out and talking to another parent in the waiting room at the doctor's office who seems to be struggling. For others, it may be joining an advocacy group and taking a leadership role in fighting for change.

At this moment in your life it may seem overwhelming to even think about giving back, as it takes all your energy to just get through the days. That's OK. At some point your child will turn a corner, have some of the support you've been fighting for, and you will have some time to breathe. Admittedly for some parents this may just be enough time to put your head above water and gasp for air. For others, it will provide the space you need to reflect on how far you and your child have come on your shared journey and you are able to plan for the road ahead.

When you do have the time to reflect, think about how you can help others. Is there any particular struggle your child has overcome with lessons learned that other caregivers could benefit from hearing about? How can you share this information? Is it through writing an email to a local or national support group outlining the struggle and how you worked to help overcome an obstacle? Is it talking to other parents who are going down the same road? Speaking at a conference? Or is it by joining a broader movement?

My first step in giving back was when my son was three months old, long before we knew about many of his challenges.

I had spent six weeks on hospital-based bed rest when I was pregnant with my son and another two weeks in the neonatal intensive care unit (NICU) with him after he was born. During my time at this large teaching hospital, I became friends with a number of medical staff. I also shared many of my observations as a patient on bed rest with my obstetrician (OB). This included the time of day routine medical tests were conducted, how complex information was relayed to moms, how the doctors could simplify their language so as to not overwhelm and confuse already stressed moms, and other observations from the bed.

Prior to my being discharged my OB asked if I would sit as a patient advocate on the perinatal council, a decision-making group made up of medical staff from antenatal, labor and delivery, as well as the NICU. While this group had no shortage of doctors, midwives, and nurses, it was lacking the voice and perspective of a patient.

I happily joined, as I am always willing to give my opinion. This committee was my first step in what has been a long road of patient advocacy. At first it was a bit overwhelming being the only nonmedical voice on a medical committee. However, I soon found my groove and looked for opportunities to not only share the patient perspective but also advocate for moms, caregivers, and the babies of the NICU.

I helped the group remember that the moms and caregivers they are working with are often sleep deprived, highly emotional, and scared. While the information being relayed may seem rational to a doctor or nurse who fully understands what is being said, it can confuse, overwhelm, or terrify the mom or dad who is trying to process the information on a few hours of sleep.

I was able to remind the medical team of the state of the mother and the challenges she was facing in addition to processing the information being provided. I helped them see the patient's perspective, and how by understanding this perspective they could change how they delivered information.

Most importantly, through my role as a patient advocate on a medical committee, I learned how a patient's voice can not only be heard, but actually result in true change being made in how medical staff interact with patients. I also gained insider knowledge of the struggles these individuals face on a daily basis (long hours, short staffing, changing government regulations, an aging workforce, and complex patient needs).

I learned that being a patient advocate involved understanding all sides of a challenge. It's not about getting angry, shouting, or blaming, but rather about having conversations and listening to the other side of the story. Often medical staff is equally frustrated about a particular roadblock, and are the messenger not the culprit. By having a calm conversation it can open up opportunities to work together on either removing the obstacle or advocating for change.

My work on the perinatal council gave me the confidence to continue on my road of patient advocacy. It gave me the tools for the battle as I had a better understanding and appreciation for the medical system.

When my son's challenges began unfolding, I knew the language needed and resources available to fight for him. I had seen how screaming and shouting only alienated caregivers, which in the long run did not help the child, only shuffled the child along to someone else in the system.

I have also been able to clearly see the role I need to play as a mother in advocating for my child. Yes, I need to fight for him, but I need to do it in a respectful and thoughtful way that will ensure I'm seen as an equal part of his medical support team versus an obstacle that needs to be avoided.

My advice to you is to find your own way to give back — no matter how big or small. Is there a parent you see struggling that could use someone to talk to? Does your local hospital have a patient advocacy department that is looking for volunteers to sit on committees? Is there a blog where you can share your story?

Giving back is an important way in not only helping remove obstacles for other caregivers but also a way to help you find the silver lining in a sometimes challenging journey. If the work you've done and lessons learned can truly help another caregiver avoid some of the same stress and frustration, it will make you realize it wasn't all in vain.

1. The Value of the Positive

In my role as a volunteer patient advocate at our local health network, I was approached to speak at a national conference for staff working in emergency departments. The coordinator was aware of my history not only as a patient advocate, but also as a conference speaker.

When he first approached me to speak, I ran through the numerous visits we as a family had had over the years to the emergency room (ER). I thought of the negative ones, the horrible ones, the neutral experiences, and the great experiences. For some reason, I thought the coordinator would want me to speak about a negative experience. After all, there were lots of lessons to be learned about what not to do in the ER to treat a child.

Before focusing on my worst experience ever, I decided to share two experiences with the conference coordinator and let him choose which one would be better suited to the conference. The first experience was a situation where my son was improperly treated for dehydration, involving one doctor's visit and two ER visits in one day, ultimately resulting in a one-week admission to pediatrics. The other experience was an amazing ER visit in a horrible situation. While the reason we went to the ER was traumatic, the patient care we received was incredible.

After going through both of these experiences, the conference coordinator was quiet for a moment and said he felt I should talk about the positive experience. He said too often medical providers hear about all the things that have gone wrong. Patients are often too willing to share their horror stories but less likely to share successes. As a result, medical providers are left feeling beaten up, frustrated, and dejected.

He felt the true learnings come from hearing what a patient experience looks like when everything goes well. In our case, all the players in my child's care did their jobs. From the 911 dispatcher to the ambulance attendants who alerted the hospital of our child's condition so the doctors and nurses were awaiting our arrival in the trauma bay, to the care we received throughout our time in the ER to the specialists at the children's hospital who were reviewing our child's case remotely; everyone did their jobs. Every person involved in our child's care played his or her role as it should have been played.

Does this mean it wasn't a stressful and difficult situation? No. We still struggled with getting through the trauma. However, in this situation the care we received allowed us to focus on supporting our child emotionally rather than having to advocate for tests or procedures. We were able to play the role we needed to play, being our child's parents and focusing on providing emotional support.

When I hung up the phone with the conference coordinator I realized he had taught me a valuable lesson: The importance of focusing on the positive. He was right, there are just as many, if not more, lessons to be learned from sharing stories of a positive patient experience versus a negative.

Funny enough, the day after this phone conversation I ran into the ER doctor who had treated my child during that experience. When I told her I'd been asked to speak at a national ER conference and would be telling a story that involved the care she provided my child, she bristled. She was fully expecting me to talk about how horrible the care was or what they did wrong.

When I told her that my talk would be focused on what excellent patient care looks like and how that experience impacts the entire family, she started to tear up. I went on to say how her care, and that of the entire team, had done so much to help us through a very difficult day.

She burst into a smile and gave me a huge hug, thanking me for sharing the story with her. She said too often doctors treat patients, and then move on to the next patient, never hearing the full outcome. This ER doctor also appreciated and recognized the value of sharing positive experiences with medical providers to show them the personal impact good patient care has on the family, not just the patient. She ended our conversation saying should would sign up to attend the conference and was so proud that she played a role in our child's care.

I share this story with you so when you are advocating your remember that patient advocacy is not just about advocating when things go wrong or there are roadblocks in your child's way. Rather patient advocacy is also about sharing successes, celebrating with medical providers, and letting others know the value of a positive patient experience. Trust me, it feels way better to be standing in front of a room of people sharing a positive experience than reliving a bad experience.

I'm not saying there isn't a time or place for sharing our negative experiences. Know that it is not only OK but there is also huge value in sharing positive patient care experiences with medical providers and other caregivers.

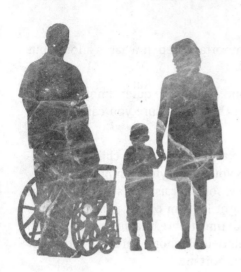

9
Final Thoughts

I hope that by reading my story and the wisdom and insights of other caregivers and medical providers, you have gained some confidence and additional tools to advocate for your child. I also hope you realize that you are not alone in this journey, and there is an entire community of caregivers and medical providers who are walking alongside you.

As roadblocks appear, take a moment to assess your energy level and decide if this is a roadblock you are prepared to tackle. If you are not emotionally or physically able to tackle this roadblock, don't beat yourself up. It might be better to conserve your energy for future challenges. If you do have the energy, then take a step back and try to analyze the roadblock and determine the tools you will need to remove or minimize it. Who from your personal support team and your child's medical team can you call on to help you? How have other caregivers approached removing or minimizing a similar roadblock? How can you best support your child?

You already have many of the tools you need to support your child. Often, the missing piece is finding and connecting with other people who can bring additional tools to help you and your child.

Just by taking the time to read this book you have already shown your commitment to supporting your child as well as improving your patient advocacy skills. This is an important step in what is a long, but meaningful journey with your child.

Please remember you aren't alone. During the quiet times, work on growing your support network and then make sure you call on them during the difficult times.

Most importantly, take the time to celebrate your child's successes, big and small. Remember while you are playing a supporting role, this is ultimately your child's journey. You are raising a strong, resilient child who not only needs you to fight for him or her, but also needs unconditional love and support. Take time to breathe and connect with this incredible child so you are reminded of whom you are fighting for and why your advocacy work is so important.

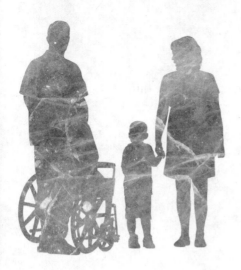

Download Kit

Please enter the URL you see in the box below into a web browser on your computer to access and use the download kit.

www.self-counsel.com/updates/ycvoice/18kit.htm

The following files are included on the download kit:

- Looking at the Big Picture
- Questions to Ask Your Case Manager
- Setting up Your Medical Team
- Developing the Case for an Educational Assistant/ Teaching Assistant or Additional Support
- Asking for Help
- Finding a Therapy Fit for Your Child
- Annual Review
- Resources

Other Titles of Interest from Self-Counsel Press

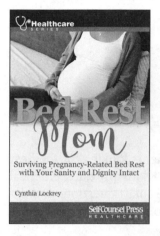

Bed Rest Mom:
Surviving Pregnancy-Related Bed Rest with Your Sanity and Dignity Intact

Cynthia Lockrey

ISBN 978-1-77040-301-7

6 x 9 • paper • 160 pp.

First Edition

$15.95 USD/$18.95 CAD

Bed rest orders may have snuck up on you, but that doesn't have to mean months of agonizing, boring time wasting, and feeling like you have lost all independence under house (or hospital) arrest as you await the arrival of your bundle of joy.

Bed Rest Mom covers the differences between what you're allowed to do (or not do) on home-based bed rest versus hospital-based bed rest. With the guidance in this book, you can decide what questions you need to ask your medical team so you can learn what to expect and make a plan to —

- stock up on snacks and proper food for the day,
- stay entertained,
- get enough sleep and appropriate exercise, and
- accomplish simple projects.

Author Cynthia Lockrey had the unique experience of enduring two high-risk pregnancies, with 19 weeks of home-based bed rest and 7 weeks of hospital-based bed rest. Her real-life experiences are weaved throughout the book in a friendly and relatable style comforting to readers.

Perhaps most important, *Bed Rest Mom* includes others' stories, so that you'll know you're not alone as you learn to deal with the "mom guilt" that often accompanies this emotionally and physically challenging time. You'll also learn ways to ask for much-needed help and support to get you through it all.

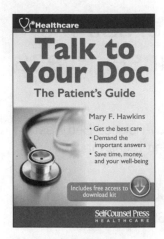

Talk to Your Doc:
The Patient's Guide

Mary F. Hawkins

ISBN 978-1-77040-227-0

6 x 9 • paper + download kit • 184 pp.

First Edition

$19.95 USD/CAD

Talk to Your Doc is the definitive guide for patients looking for the best possible health outcome. Author Mary F. Hawkins provides practical communication strategies to help you ask the smart questions and develop the best relationship with health-care providers and the health-care system.

Remember, doctors are busier than ever, so your time with them has to be well-spent. *Talk to Your Doc* helps you develop a clear strategy to get the right treatment with the right approach to caring for yourself and for your loved ones. It also takes the stress out of the challenges of dealing with doctors and institutions.

There is more information than ever available for patients, but sorting through it requires professional help. Mary provides this help in *Talk to your Doc*. This book builds confidence in our most vulnerable situations.

About the author

Mary F. Hawkins has been an author on medicine and health communications, a health-care columnist, a University of Ottawa Communications Lecturer since 1998, and a photojournalist, as well as working in the media as a producer, broadcast researcher, and sometimes on-air. She has been an extensive public speaker and commentator. She lives in Ottawa.